T0146804

DIABETES

Also by Susan Weiner
The Complete Diabetes Organizer: Your Guide to a
Less Stressful and More Manageable Diabetes Life

Also by Paula Ford-Martin
The Everything Health Guide to Diabetes
The Everything Health Guide to Type 2 Diabetes
The Everything Pregnancy Book
The Everything Pregnancy Organizer
The Only Pregnancy Book You'll Ever Need

DIABETES

365

TIPS FOR LIVING WELL

Susan Weiner, MS, RDN, CDE, CDN
Paula Ford-Martin

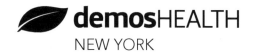

demosHEALTH

NEW YORK

Visit our website at www.demoshealth.com

ISBN: 978-1-936303-91-5
e-book ISBN: 978-1-61705-258-3

Acquisitions Editor: Julia Pastore
Compositor: diacriTech

Medical information provided by Demos Health, in the absence of a visit with a health care professional, must be considered as an educational service only. This book is not designed to replace a physician's independent judgment about the appropriateness or risks of a procedure or therapy for a given patient. Our purpose is to provide you with information that will help you make your own health care decisions.

The information and opinions provided here are believed to be accurate and sound, based on the best judgment available to the authors, editors, and publisher, but readers who fail to consult appropriate health authorities assume the risk of injuries. The publisher is not responsible for errors or omissions. The editors and publisher welcome any reader to report to the publisher any discrepancies or inaccuracies noticed.

Library of Congress Cataloging-in-Publication Data
Weiner, Susan.
Diabetes : 365 tips for living well / Susan Weiner and Paula Ford-Martin.
    pages cm
 Includes bibliographical references and index.
 ISBN 978-1-936303-91-5
 1. Diabetes — Popular works. I. Ford-Martin, Paula. II. Title.
RC660.4.W45 2015
616.4'62 — dc23

2015015134

Special discounts on bulk quantities of Demos Health books are available to corporations, professional associations, pharmaceutical companies, health care organizations, and other qualifying groups. For details, please contact:

Special Sales Department
Demos Medical Publishing, LLC
11 West 42nd Street, 15th Floor
New York, NY 10036
Phone: 800-532-8663 or 212-683-0072
Fax: 212-941-7842
E-mail: specialsales@demosmedical.com

Printed in the United States of America by McNaughton & Gunn.
15 16 17 18 19 / 5 4 3 2 1

To my best friends and confidants: my mom, Marcia Greenberg, and my sister, Jill Greenberg-Halman.

—Susan Weiner

For my husband Tim, the love of my life and the truest man I know.

—Paula Ford Martin

Contents

Foreword

I met Paula Ford-Martin and Susan Weiner in 2004 when I started working at dLifeTV, a television show created for *and by* people with diabetes. Paula and Susan were a couple of the handful of people who worked there who did not have diabetes.

When we began shooting dLifeTV, I had lugged around this persistent and overwhelming disease (type 1 diabetes) for 33 years. In those 33 years I'd somehow, mistakenly, come to believe that I knew everything about diabetes. In reality, the "everything" I knew about diabetes would better be defined as "street smarts." But much of my "street-smart" wisdom wasn't really very smart at all, and some part of that "everything" weren't even things. It was just stuff I'd made up over the years to fit my idea of how to manage this complicated disease.

Suddenly, I was surrounded by people who studied and were all learned and what-have-you about diabetes, and even though many of them didn't have to lug the beast around, they knew lots and lots of *actual stuff* about the disease. Paula and Susan were at the top of that list. They each became my go-to about all things diabetes.

Wayyyy back when I was diagnosed in 1970, there were only a couple of books about diabetes. The *Joslin Guide to Diabetes* was the one I read and reread and reread looking for any clues at all about how to manage the unwieldy beast living inside me. Back then, actual control seemed out of grasp. I just corralled it and tried hard not to get kicked in the head. We didn't have blood sugar meters, insulin pumps, A1C tests, constant glucose monitors, and so on. So says grandpa.

We were flying blind. Diabetes management—mine anyway—was by "feel."

Things are so different—and better—now. We have all those things and much, much more. Finally, today we have tools to fight—or rather, *live with*—this disease. We have so many tools that it's actually kind of daunting and sometimes overwhelming.

Working with Susan and Paula over the years, I have picked up countless tips and ideas about control of this perplexing disease. And even though I was the one who had lugged it around for 33 years to that point (right now I'm at 44 years, 359 days, 16 hours and 44 minutes—but who's counting?) it was they who would often point the way out of trouble.

When it comes to my life, and especially my diabetes, I don't like things complicated and I don't like to get overwhelmed. Diabetes is complicated and overwhelming enough. I like simple, straightforward suggestions.

Here's a year of them.

One at a time.

The way it should be.

When Susan and Paula told me their idea for this book, a little voice in the back of my head screamed at me. "JIM! Why didn't *you* think of that?"

It's just so obviously brilliant. What was I doing while they were coming up with this?

One simple, straightforward tip every single day … Genius.

I hope that with this book Susan and Paula give that overwhelmingness a bit of a whooping. In fact, I hope that they will give it a good old-fashioned boot stomping.

And I have to say, I am honored that they asked me to write the Foreword to this wonderful book. But honestly, I can't stop thinking, what if I …

Jim Turner

Jim Turner has appeared in countless television, film, and live theater roles. You may know him from his lead role in *Arli$$* (HBO), as Randee of the Redwoods (MTV), or from his more recent appearances in *The Big Bang Theory* and *Parenthood*. Jim was diagnosed with type 1 diabetes as a teenager in 1970, and shares his experiences in his one-man live show, *Diabetes: My Struggles With Jim Turner*.

January

January is a time of new beginnings and a chance to start the New Year off fresh with healthy habits and goals. This month we focus on tips that help you reset old behaviors, try new things, and set yourself up for a successful year of living well with diabetes.

1 Ring In the New Year Right

Too many New Year's resolutions go off the rails by the end of January. Why? Usually it's because they are too vague, too grand in scale, or too unrealistic. This year, make a single resolution: to make an effort to improve your diabetes health. Spend an hour making a thoughtful list of things you think you can do better, such as testing your blood sugar, eating right, or moving more. Once you've done this, you're ready to set some goals.

2 Make SMART Goals for the Year

Once you have a list of health goals for the year, make it SMART. That means it should be Specific, Measurable, Action Oriented, Realistic, and Timely. Instead of "lower my A1C three points," a SMART goal would be, "I will start walking one mile, at least three times a week, and test my blood sugar before and after." Goals can and should change as the year progresses. Focusing on one at a time increases your chances of making them permanent habits.

3 Think Small

It may sound counterintuitive, but when you are setting a weight loss goal, think small. Studies show that a loss of as little as 2 to 5 percent of your total body weight can do big things for your health, such as improving blood sugar and blood pressure control. And a small weight loss goal is both easier to achieve and meets all the criteria of SMART goals.

4 Get Moving

You've heard it before, but we'll say it again—any amount of additional activity helps improve your health. You don't need to run a marathon (unless you really want to … then, more power to you). Just make a small, realistic commitment to a little more movement each week. Sign up for a dance class. Walk the dog. Meet a friend for coffee and walk around the mall.

5 Remember to Take Your Meds

Have trouble remembering to take your daily medicines? Here are a few ideas that may help. Use a daily pill organizer that you fill once a week on the same day. Keep it in the same, highly visible spot all the time (near the coffee maker works for some people). Try setting an alarm on your watch or smartphone to remind you when to take your pills. Finally, automate all refills with your pharmacy and/ or mail-order company.

6 Veggies in Season: Greens

Greens, such as spinach, kale, and collards, are in abundance during the winter months. They are also very low in carbs and calories and high in nutrients—a winning combination for people with diabetes. All three can be cooked, but in their raw form they have more nutrients and make a great salad base. Collards and kale are tougher than traditional salad greens, so try dressing them with oil and vinegar first to soften them up for a great tasting salad.

7 Dialog With Your Doctor

When you go to your next diabetes care appointment, be prepared. Keep a running list of questions that come up between appointments, and bring it with you. Sometimes it's helpful to bring a spouse or significant other as support (and another set of ears). Do not be afraid to ask questions if you don't understand something.

8 Fill Up on Fiber

Fiber can help us feel fuller longer. Soluble fiber regulates blood sugar by signaling the liver to stop making glucose and improving insulin sensitivity. It also lowers "bad" cholesterol or low-density lipoprotein (LDL). Sources of soluble fiber include oats, beans, apples, citrus fruits, and carrots. Insoluble-fiber prevents constipation and may also help control blood sugar. Good sources include wheat, corn, nuts, and dark green leafy vegetables. Get plenty of both!

9 Write Down Every Bite

Writing down everything you eat in a food diary or journal (or a food tracking app) is a great way to stay accountable. It's also helpful to include the time you're eating and your feelings while eating (such as stress, boredom, or anxiety). Food journals can help identify nutritional issues as well as emotional and behavioral responses to daily situations. They make us practice "mindful eating."

10 Cutting Calories for Weight Loss

Drastic calorie reductions can actually hinder weight loss efforts by triggering hormonal changes that promote weight gain. If you have a large amount of weight to lose, cutting back by just a few hundred calories—and sticking to nutrient-dense, lower carbohydrate food choices—is your best bet for successfully losing the weight and keeping it off.

11 Portions in the Palm of Your Hand

Because restaurant and fast-food portions have grown substantially over the past few decades, many Americans have internalized this "super sizing" as normal. They are shocked when they learn a single portion of beef should really only be the size of a deck of cards, and a pasta portion about the size of a tennis ball. Here is an easy way to establish real portions with a reference guide you always have with you—your hands.

| 1 teaspoon | 1 tablespoon | 1 ounce | 3 ounces | 1/2 cup | 1 cup |

12 Exercising Through Injury

Exercise is a critical tool for blood sugar control, but injuries can present a major roadblock. It's important to find safe ways to keep yourself moving during your recovery. Swimming is a good low-impact option for people recovering from injury or joint replacement. If you have an orthopedic injury, your physical therapist may prescribe a regimen of specific exercises. Do them regularly and they will help you heal faster.

13 Exercise for Everyone

Do you have joint problems, limited mobility, or other chronic health issues that make regular exercise difficult? Expand your idea of what exercise really is. Chair workouts are an excellent alternative. They allow you to exercise the parts of your body you can at a safe level, and they offer you stability for the workout.

14 Frozen

If you have diabetic peripheral neuropathy (DPN, or nerve damage), it's important to bundle up when braving the elements this winter. Why? The stinging, burning, and numbness that signals the onset of frostbite are the same exact set of symptoms that people with DPN feel in their hands and feet. Which means that you may not feel any danger signs of frostbite until it's too late.

15 Diabetes Winter Skin Care

Dry, cracked skin is a breeding ground for infection and skin wounds, and if you have diabetes you are at higher risk for both. In winter, when the air is dry and so is your skin, use body lotion regularly, run a humidifier in your home, and drink plenty of water each day to keep your skin smooth and supple.

16 When to Test

Testing your blood sugar at home is the best way to tell how different foods and activities impact your levels. A postprandial test is a blood sugar check you do after meals. You should do this test from one to two hours after the start of your meal, as this is the time when blood sugar spikes highest after eating. Speak with your doctor or diabetes educator and make sure you understand when you should be testing each day.

17 Rate Your Hunger

The next time you are standing in front of an open refrigerator or pantry and you aren't actively cooking a meal, take a moment to check in with yourself. Are you truly hungry? We often grab food out of boredom or habit, mistaking it for hunger. Or we "self-medicate" with food when we're feeling bad. Understanding why we eat when we aren't hungry is the first step in developing healthier behaviors.

18 January Fruit Fact

If life hands you lemons this month, you can be happy about it. In addition to being full of fiber and vitamin C, lemon juice has a low glycemic index and can blunt postprandial (after meal) blood sugar spikes. Of course lemons are a bit too sour to just bite into and enjoy for most people, but in slices or as juice they add great flavor and a tart bite to salad dressings, beverages, seafood, and poultry.

19 It's All About the Carbs

Although other nutrients, such as fat and protein, do play a role in our dietary health, for people with diabetes it's the "total carbohydrate" in a food that has the biggest impact on raising blood sugar. Always check this value on the labels of the foods you buy. When you grocery shop and plan your meals, consider that an entire meal should be around 45 grams of carbohydrates (potentially less, depending on your specific needs).

20 The Mouth-Diabetes Connection

Uncontrolled diabetes increases the risk for bacterial and fungal growth in your mouth and can cause damage to your teeth and gums. Recent research has found a connection between periodontal (gum) problems and cardiovascular disease. Keep your mouth and heart healthy through good blood sugar control, and by brushing your teeth at least twice a day, and flossing at least once daily. Visit your dentist at least twice a year for cleanings and a thorough checkup.

21 Keep Your Mouth Moist

High blood sugars can make your mouth dry. Even if your blood sugar is usually in range, there are many prescription and over-the-counter medicines that have dry mouth, also known as *xerostomia*, as a side effect. Sip water throughout the day, and try sugar-free gum to keep the saliva flowing. Dry mouth can also contribute to chapped lips, so use lip balm frequently, especially in the winter months.

22 Drink More Water

Water is good for you. It raises your metabolic rate and therefore helps with weight control. It's also a great thirst quencher that will keep you well-hydrated and can replace high-calorie, high-carbohydrate drinks such as soda, sugary juices, and alcohol. You should drink at least 48 ounces of water a day. But if you have kidney disease, please, make sure to discuss your water consumption with your doctor.

23 Clean Out Your Medicine Cabinet

Do you know what's in your medicine cabinet? Take everything out of the cabinet. Check expiration dates, and throw away everything that is past its prime or that you no longer use or need (some medicines may need special disposal; ask your pharmacist if you aren't sure). Blood sugar testing strips and ketone strips should be kept in a dry environment, so if your medicine cabinet is in a bathroom with a shower, these supplies should be moved to a less humid location.

24 Use Your Plate to Plan

Divide your plate in two. Fill one half with nonstarchy vegetables (e.g., broccoli, cauliflower, salad greens). High in fiber and nutrients and low in carbs, these veggies should make up half of your meal. On the other half of the plate are foods that should be eaten in smaller portions. One quarter of the plate should have a lean protein (e.g., fish, poultry) and the final quarter contains a starch (e.g., whole grain bread, quinoa, sweet potato).

25 Watch Expiration Dates: Glucagon

Glucagon, a drug used to treat a severe low blood sugar, is a prescription that everyone who takes insulin should have on hand. Fortunately, you may not need to use it. But like all medicines, it carries an expiration date and will lose potency after that date. Know when your glucagon expires and get it refilled before that date.

26 Watch Expiration Dates: Test Strips

The test strips you use to check your blood sugar at home also carry expiration dates. Expired strips can produce inaccurate results, so it's important to keep track of this date. If you pick up test strips at the pharmacy, it's a good practice to check the date before you leave the store. If the date doesn't seem far enough in the future, ask for a newer package.

27 Is It Your Thyroid?

January is Thyroid Awareness Month. Hypothyroidism is the most common thyroid problem in people with diabetes, and it can make your blood sugar harder to control. Unfortunately, many of its symptoms, such as weight gain, fatigue, and depression, may be attributed to your diabetes and go untreated. Ask your doctor about getting your thyroid hormone levels tested.

28 Visit a Registered Dietitian Nutritionist/ Certified Diabetes Educator

If you have never seen a registered dietitian nutritionist, it's time to make an appointment. A registered dietitian nutritionist (RDN) will work with you to create a customized eating plan that fits your lifestyle. She will also work with you to set and achieve health goals. Choose an RDN who is also a certified diabetes educator (CDE), as these professionals have deep expertise in diabetes treatment and can better address your unique dietary needs.

29 Eat Often

People with diabetes should try to eat five to six times each day. Spacing out your food will help to stabilize your blood sugar and control hunger. It will also keep you from overeating when you feel like you are "starving."

30 Count Snack Carbs

A good rule of thumb is keeping carbs at around 45 grams for a meal and less than 15 grams for a snack; however, everyone has different goals (an RDN/CDE can help you figure out yours). As you start off each week, take the time to portion your favorite snacks in baggies or containers and label them with the carbohydrate count. Then group them together in a bin so you can locate a "carb-counted" snack when you need one.

31 The Scoop on Stevia

Stevia is a noncaloric, zero carbohydrate sweetener made from a South American plant. It is much sweeter than sugar, and also sweeter than earlier entries to the sugar substitute market such as sucralose, aspartame, and saccharin. Despite the extreme sweetness, some people prefer it as a more "natural" alternative to those products. If you are new to stevia, we suggest that you start with a very small amount and work your way up to a preferred level of sweetness.

February

Take this month to heart. Not only is February a time of roses, romance, and chocolate, but it's also American Heart Month. Since people with diabetes have a higher risk of heart attack and cardio-vascular disease, it's important to focus on healthy heart habits. Stay healthy and loved with these February tips.

1. Super Bowl Sunday

Before America's biggest game this month, follow a few simple tips to stay on track with your diabetes control. To avoid bingeing on party foods, don't starve yourself before game time. Drink plenty of water to keep alcohol consumption down and to feel full. And finally, get strategic with your snacking. Don't eat directly from a bag of chips or sit at the snack table. If you plate your portions you'll be more mindful of what you eat.

2. Deep Freeze

If you live in the North, February can be a hard month. Snow and ice can prevent regular outdoor exercise, and blood sugar management can suffer as a result. Of course there's always the gym, if there's one nearby that fits your personal and financial needs. If not, you do have other choices. Walk an indoor mall. Swim inside at a community center. You can even rent or buy an exercise game for your kid's gaming station so you can Zumba in your living room.

3. Bundle Up Your Blood Sugar Meter

Freezing temperatures can affect the accuracy of your blood sugar testing supplies. If you are braving the elements outdoors for skiing or snowman building, make sure your meter and strips stay warm by storing them in an insulated bag. The same goes for insulin: frozen insulin is ineffective insulin.

4. Cauliflower Comfort Foods

Try swapping starchy, high glycemic potatoes for lower carb cauliflower in your favorite potato dishes. Mashed cauliflower, broiled cauliflower, and cauliflower "potato" salad—the possibilities are endless. If you aren't sure about the taste, try mixing half potato and half cauliflower until you adjust your tastebuds.

5 Veggies in Season: Brussels Sprouts

Forget the bad rap Brussels sprouts get. These versatile veggies are packed with vitamin C, fiber, and folate. And roasted, steamed, grilled, or stir-fried, they are a delicious addition to any February meal and have just 8 grams of carbohydrates (and over 3 grams of fiber) per cup. Try some for dinner tonight!

6 Stop Smoking for Your Heart

If you smoke, stop. It's the best thing you can do to protect your cardiovascular system, which is already at risk for problems in people with diabetes. In addition to all the other health problems smoking can cause, the nicotine in cigarettes narrows your blood vessels, driving up blood pressure and increasing your heart attack risk. Talk to your doctor about a smoking cessation program, and do it today.

7 Count Your Snack Carbs

Don't forget to count your snack carbs. Aim for about 15 grams of carbohydrates per snack. Once or twice a week, take some time to preproportion snacks in baggies or reusable plastic containers and store them in your fridge and pantry. When between-meal hunger strikes, you'll have a carb-smart snack solution at your fingertips.

8 Smart Snack Ideas

Need some new snack ideas that won't break the carb bank? Try one of these: half an apple with 2 tablespoons of natural peanut butter, ¾ of a cup of blueberries, 3 tablespoons of hummus with 1 cup of baby carrots, or 3 cups of air-popped popcorn. All have about 15 grams of carbohydrates.

9 Shake the Salt Habit

Just 1 teaspoon of table salt contains 2,400 milligrams of sodium. That is more than a full day's worth of sodium for anyone trying to follow a low-sodium diet to control their blood pressure. Stow your saltshaker and try one of the many sodium-free spice blends available at your local grocery store. You may find you like them more than salt when it comes to adding flavor to your favorite foods.

10 Just Desserts for Your Heart

The cocoa bean (also called cacao) is rich in flavonoids that fight heart disease. Dark chocolate is highest in flavonoids. When reading labels, look for a high percentage of cocoa and steer clear of anything that says "dutch processed" or "alkalinization," as this reduces the health benefits.

11 Sex and Diabetes: Your Body

Diabetes can affect your sex life in many different ways. Nerve damage and circulation problems can cause arousal problems in both men and women. They can also impact performance even if you can achieve arousal. The good news is that, like most things in life with diabetes, working with your doctor to get a handle on your blood sugar control can help improve these diabetic complications (along with appropriate treatment).

12 Sex and Diabetes: Your Mind

Depression is very common in people with diabetes, and this often has an impact on your intimate relationships. So does all the other emotional baggage that can accompany diabetes (e.g., guilt, anxiety, poor self-image). Since sex involves the brain just as much as the body, sometimes these bad feelings end up affecting sexual arousal and function. A good therapist can help you work through these issues.

13 Sex and Diabetes: Getting Help

If you are having problems getting or staying aroused in the bedroom, you need to talk to your doctor. Get over any embarrassment you might have. Your doctor has heard this same question at least 100 times before, and many treatment options for both men and women are now available. Don't delay the discussion any longer—you and your partner deserve a healthy and happy sex life.

14 Happy Valentine's Day

If you have a spouse or significant other, today is a good day to think about the role he plays in your diabetes life. If he is already supportive, make sure he knows how much you appreciate the role he plays. If you could use a little more back up, ask him to come to a diabetes education class with you. It's a great way for your partner to understand more about diabetes and get perspective from others.

15 Dating With Diabetes: Safety First

If you are out in the dating world, you may struggle with how and when to tell a new companion you have diabetes. If your date doesn't yet know about your diabetes, make sure that you wear your medical ID in case of emergency. And observe "dating safety" rules that everyone should practice, such as letting family or friends know who you are heading out with and going to a public place for a first meeting.

16 Testing Tip: Getting a Good Blood Sample

If you have trouble getting a large enough finger-stick blood sample for testing, try these techniques. Rub your hands together briskly to warm them up and get the circulation going. Or try shaking them at your sides, below heart level, to get your blood flowing. It's also OK to squeeze your finger to get an adequate blood drop; this won't affect your blood sugar reading.

17 Supply Storage: Expiration Dates

When you get a new box of diabetes supplies or medication, check the expiration date. When you store it with other supplies, make sure the closest date is at the front of the shelf, drawer, or cabinet. This way your oldest supplies are up front and will be used first before they expire.

18 Fruits in Season: Prickly Pears

Prickly pears are the fruit of the nopal cactus. They are packed with fiber, vitamin C, and antioxidants. They may also help improve cholesterol and blood sugar levels. This South American delicacy is imported to the United States in the winter season and is available in food markets and some grocery stores. Just peel carefully (they are prickly, after all) and enjoy!

19 Heart Attack in Women: Know the Signs

Women with diabetes have an increased risk of heart attack. But the symptoms won't always be simple chest pain. Know what to look for. Shortness of breath, nausea, dizziness, and extreme fatigue are all potential signs of heart attack in women. You may also have arm, back, neck, jaw, or stomach pain. Although some women may experience pain and pressure in their chests, not all do.

20 Add Omega-3s

Omega-3s are important because they can lower blood pressure and LDL (bad) cholesterol, reduce inflammation, and protect against heart disease—all important considerations for people with diabetes. As with most nutrients, the best way to get omega-3s is through your food. So eat more fatty fish (e.g., salmon, tuna), walnuts, wheat germ, and ground flaxseed, and cook with canola or soybean vegetable oils.

21 Fresh, Frozen, or Canned?

What's the best choice for fruits and veggies—fresh, frozen, or canned? Fresh may have the most nutrients most of the time, but seasonality, cost, accessibility, and convenience are all factors in what you choose at the grocery store. First and foremost, buy what you will use and eat. One caveat—canned veggies and fruits can have added salt and sugar, so do try low sodium and sugar-free versions, or rinse them before preparing.

22 Diabetes at Work: Know Your Rights

Did you know that federal law requires employers with 15 or more employees to provide you with "reasonable accommodations" to care for your diabetes on the job? For example, giving you breaks to check blood sugar levels. If your employer isn't accommodating your diabetes needs, contact the American Diabetes Association at 1-800-DIABETES (800-342-2383) for help.

23 Diabetes at Work: Do I Tell Coworkers?

You have no legal obligation to inform anyone at your workplace that you have diabetes. But your boss will need to know if you are requesting reasonable accommodations to care for yourself at work. And from a safety perspective, sharing with your supervisor or other close coworkers is a good idea in case you need their help in an emergency. If you do not disclose, it's even more important to wear a medical ID.

24 Neuropathy and Your Skin

Neuropathy, or nerve damage, is one of the most common complications of diabetes. In addition to discomfort, such as numbness, tingling, and burning, neuropathy can also cause a decrease in skin moisture. If you have diabetic neuropathy, make sure you use moisturizer.

25 Nutrition Label Hot Spots

Know your nutrition hot spots—those areas on the nutrition facts food label that can have the biggest impact on your diabetes health. The "Total Carbs" in a food is the most important indicator of how it will affect your blood sugar.

Foods high in "Dietary Fiber" digest more slowly and help blunt blood sugar impact. Finally, consider the "Serving Size," because what is listed is often dramatically different from what people actually eat.

Current

Nutrition Facts

Serving Size 1 cup (228g)
Servings Per Container about 2

Amount Per Serving

Calories 250   Calories from Fat 110

	% Daily Value*
Total Fat 12g	18%
Saturated Fat 3g	15%
Trans Fat 3g	
Cholesterol 30mg	10%
Sodium 470mg	20%
Total Carbohydrate 31g	10%
Dietary Fiber 0g	0%
Sugars 5g	
Proteins 5g	
Vitamin A	4%
Vitamin C	2%
Calcium	20%
Iron	4%

* Percent Daily Values are based on a 2,000 calorie diet. Your Daily Values may be higher or lower depending on your calorie needs:

	Calories:	2,000	2,500
Total Fat	Less than	65g	80g
Saturated Fat	Less than	20g	25g
Cholesterol	Less than	300mg	300mg
Sodium	Less than	2,400mg	2,400mg
Total Carbohydrate		300g	375g
Dietary Fiber		25g	30g

For educational purposes only. This label does not meet the labeling requirements described in 21 CFR 101.9.

Proposed Alternate

Nutrition Facts

8 servings per container

Serving size   2/3 cup (55g)

Amount per 2/3 cup

Calories   **230**

% Daily Value*

QUICK FACTS:

12%	**Total Fat** 8g
12%	**Total Carbs** 37g
	Sugars 1g
	Protein 3g

AVOID TOO MUCH:

5%	Saturated Fat 1g
	Trans Fat 0g
0%	**Cholesterol** 0mg
7%	**Sodium** 160mg
	Added Sugars 0g

GET ENOUGH:

14%	Fiber 4g
10%	Vitamin D 2mcg
20%	Calcium 260mg
45%	Iron 8mg
5%	Potassium 235mg

* Footnote on Daily Values (DV) and calorie reference to be inserted here.

26 The Dreaded "E" Word

Exercise is critical to managing blood sugar levels, protecting heart health, and increasing insulin sensitivity in people with diabetes. Yet many of us continue to avoid it—"it's hard work" or "it's boring" are frequent excuses. Here's a lifesaving tip for you—it doesn't have to be either. Hate the gym? Don't go! Do something you love, such as hiking, dog walking, or gardening. The only criteria are that it gets you moving and that you like it (making it much more likely that you'll stick to it).

27 Dance for Diabetes

If you love music and have even the slightest sense of rhythm, dancing is a great workout. The best part? It's both a solo and group activity, so if you're shy, start slow at home. If you're social, join a class or go out on the town. Above all, have fun and keep at it.

28 Always Eat Breakfast

It really is the most important meal of the day. So start it off right with some protein to promote fullness without raising blood sugar. Among traditional breakfast foods, you can include eggs, cheese, plain Greek yogurt, and natural nut butter. You can also add in some healthy fiber in the form of steel cut oats or a high-fiber cereal with a handful of almonds and berries.

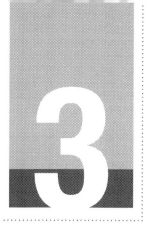

March

Even though Spring is on its way, cold and flu season lingers on this month. Make sure you take good care of yourself by managing illness, eating well, and exercising regularly. Whether March comes in like a lion or a lamb, follow this month's tips to spring into better diabetes control.

1 Surviving Sick Days

When you are sick or injured, you need to pay close attention to your blood sugar levels. Illness can cause blood sugar to rise. You may need to adjust your medication to compensate. And if you are vomiting, that can cause even bigger problems with blood sugar control. At your next diabetes appointment, talk to your doctor about a sick-day plan—a written set of instructions to follow when you are feeling under the weather.

2 Ketone Testing

Have a bottle of ketone testing strips on hand at home. Ketones are produced when your body burns fat for energy, and they can make you very sick in large amounts. These are especially important for sick days; when you are ill, ketone levels can increase to dangerous levels. If your blood sugar is over 250 mg/dL for two or more tests, check your ketone levels. Call your doctor if they are high.

3 Cold Medicines and Your Blood Sugar

Before you buy over-the-counter (OTC) medicine for a bad cold, check in with the pharmacist. Many OTC medicines can raise your blood sugar levels. Tell your pharmacist you have diabetes and ask what cold remedies you can use that won't raise your blood sugar.

4 Are You SURE That's Diet Soda?

Here's a neat trick to help you ensure that the diet soda you ordered is in fact diet. Keep a vial of urine (not blood) glucose test strips in your bag. When your drink comes, put a drop of soda on a test strip. If the strip changes color, your soda is not sugar free. Different brands of strips work differently, so read the directions for use first.

5 Eat With Purpose

Turn off the TV during meals, and stay away from big bags of snack food while playing a game or watching a movie. Studies show that people who eat while distracted eat past the point of satiety, or fullness, and consume excess calories. That can lead to weight gain and problems with diabetes control.

6 Veggies in Season: Asparagus

It's National Nutrition Month! Pick up some asparagus for a plate full of fiber, protein, folate, and vitamins A, C, E, and K. Six medium asparagus spears contain just 3 grams of carbohydrates. Try roasting them or grilling with a drizzle of olive oil and minced garlic.

7 Keep Your Kidneys Healthy

March is National Kidney Month, and a good time to make sure you are doing what you need to keep your kidneys healthy. At least once a year, most adults with diabetes should have a urine screening test for kidney problems. If you haven't had one in the past year, call your doctor today and ask to schedule one.

8 Know Your Blood Pressure

Controlling your blood pressure is also a critical part of keeping your kidneys healthy (as well as your cardiovascular system, eyes, and feet). Most adults with diabetes should have a blood pressure goal of less than 140/90 mmHg (your goal may vary depending on your individual health history).

9 DASH for Better Blood Pressure

The Dietary Approaches to Stop Hypertension (DASH) program is an eating plan rich in fruits, vegetables, lean protein, low-fat dairy products, and whole grains. It limits simple sugars and sodium and is rich in potassium, magnesium, calcium, and fiber. Studies show that the DASH program lowers high blood pressure and improves blood cholesterol levels. A registered dietitian nutritionist (RDN) can help you get started on a DASH program while still balancing your carbohydrate intake.

10 Nuts for Health

Nuts are very nutritious and filled with vitamins, minerals, and omega-3 fatty acids. They also pack a powerful protein punch. One ounce of almonds has just 160 calories and 6 grams of protein. One ounce of Brazil nuts has about 190 calories and 4 grams of protein. And 14 walnut halves have 190 calories and 4 grams of protein. Eat them alone or use them to top veggies or a salad.

11 Nuts for Snacks

Most nuts are low in carbohydrates, which also makes them a smart snack choice for people with diabetes. Portion control is the key; it is very easy to eat an entire bag of nuts instead of a single portion, which will overdo it on the calories. The good news is that the protein, fiber, and fat in a portion of nuts will keep you feeling fuller for longer.

12 Know the Code Names for Salt

Most Americans eat too much salt. Since sodium can raise blood pressure, this is a problem for many people with diabetes. Although avoiding added table salt isn't hard, many packaged foods contain hidden forms of sodium such as monosodium glutamate (MSG), baking soda, seasoned salts, and marinades. Look for these code names on food labels. You should also limit foods that are cured (e.g., salami, bacon), packed in brine (e.g., pickles, olives), or smoked (e.g., salmon).

13 It's OK to Indulge

Everyone deserves a treat once in a while, and that includes people with diabetes. Just follow a few simple rules. Keep portion sizes reasonable, depending on what the treat is. If a supersize piece of cake is on the dessert menu, split it with your dining companion. And be aware of the big picture. If you know you'll be having a favorite dessert at dinner, plan accordingly and scale back on other carbs in the meal.

14 Help With Heart Rate

How do you know you aren't under- or overdoing it when you exercise? Follow your heart rate. Your maximum heart rate is calculated by taking 220 minus your age. Your target heart rate zone during exercise should be 50 to 85 percent of your maximum. So if you are 50 years old, your maximum heart rate would be 170 and your target zone would be between 85 and 145. If you have a heart condition or you take blood pressure medicine, ask your doctor what your heart rate target should be.

15 Avoid Impulse Buys

Always make a detailed shopping list before you head out to the grocery store. This helps you avoid impulse buys of less healthy options. It also prevents purchases of multiple items that result in wasted food. If you buy only what you need to prepare healthy, preplanned meals, you'll save money and stay within your calorie count and budget.

16 Changing Your Lancet

A lancet is a small needle used to poke through the skin and draw blood for blood sugar tests. With each use, a lancet gets duller, and that means that finger sticks can get more painful. Lancet manufacturers recommend changing the lancet after each use, but how often you change your lancet is ultimately up to you. Just ensure that it is clean and works properly. And never share a lancet with anyone else.

17 Safe Celebrations

Happy St. Patrick's Day, a holiday second only to New Year's Eve in alcohol consumption. Stay safe by limiting alcohol to one or two drinks (two for men, one for women). Stay away from sugary cocktail mixers that can raise blood sugar. Wear your medical ID in case of emergency. And remember that drinking can cause overnight low blood sugars, so set your alarm to test several hours into your sleep for the night.

18 Fruits in Season: Oranges

Peel yourself a juicy orange as part of your diabetes-friendly meal plan. A medium navel orange is only about 70 calories and provides more than 100 percent of the daily recommended amount of vitamin C, as well as being high in fiber, folate, and potassium. It also has 18 grams of carbohydrates, making it a good choice for a between-meal snack.

19 The Power of the Peanut

March is Peanut Month, and a great time to celebrate that perennial lunchbox favorite—peanut butter. In fact, all nut and seed butters pack a powerful nutrition punch. They are naturally cholesterol free and are good sources of plant-based protein and dietary fiber. However, be wary of reduced fat versions because the fat is often replaced by extra sugar. Natural nut butters are usually best. And remember to keep portions to about a tablespoon (or 100 calories).

20 Optimizing Your Sleep Environment

Proper sleep is critical to your overall health and to keeping your diabetes under control. Adults should get seven to nine hours of sleep each night. Part of ensuring a consistent sleep pattern is making sure your bedroom is a restful environment. A healthy sleep environment should be dark, slightly cool, and free of noise and distractions. If outside light is a problem, blackout curtains may help.

21 Get Running with Diabetes

Start a running program in three simple steps. First, see your doctor or certified diabetes educator (CDE). They may have suggestions to help adjust medicine and carbohydrate intake around your runs. Second, visit your podiatrist or pedorthist to get a recommendation for the right kind of running shoe for you. Third, test to make sure your blood sugar is in the appropriate range before, during, and after your run, and always carry glucose tablets so you can treat low blood sugar if needed.

22 Are You Getting Enough Water?

March 22 is World Water Day. Getting enough water is critical to your kidney health. Studies show that high daily water intake is protective against chronic kidney disease, something people with diabetes are at a higher risk of developing. Fruits and veggies are also a great source of additional daily water intake. And remember to try to drink 48 to 64 ounces of water each day.

23 Autonomic Neuropathy

Your autonomic nervous system helps to control "involuntary" functions, such as heartbeat, digestion, and regulation of body temperature. Chronically high blood sugars can damage these nerves and cause problems with one or more of these bodily functions. There are tests you can take to determine if you have this condition, which is known as autonomic neuropathy. Ask your doctor if you should be screened.

24 Adaptive Technology for Everyone

Many people with diabetes have physical disabilities. Recognizing this, diabetes supply manufacturers have designed products that can help overcome these obstacles. There are blood sugar meters that "speak" results and those that have extra large displays for people with vision issues. People with dexterity problems can benefit from special insulin pens designed for ease of use. A CDE can help you find products that fit your needs.

25 Treating Sleep Apnea

Studies indicate that between 58 and 86 percent of people with type 2 diabetes have obstructive sleep apnea (OSA), a breathing disorder that adversely affects diabetes control and increases insulin resistance. The good news is that treating OSA with a continuous positive airway pressure (C-PAP) machine can help improve sleep quality and assist in decreasing A1C levels.

26 Ban the Working Lunch

When you work through lunch or eat at your desk, you aren't fully enjoying and experiencing your food. Research shows that people often overeat in these circumstances. If an occasional working lunch is unavoidable at your job, set yourself up for success. Plan ahead and pack a healthy, portion-controlled lunch. And take a break later to stretch your legs and move!

27 Prepping for the Hospital

If you are headed to the hospital, it pays to be prepared. Bring your blood sugar testing supplies to the hospital with you. And be proactive about guarding against hospital-acquired infections. If you haven't already gotten one, get a flu shot prior to admission. When in the hospital, make sure visitors wash their hands or use hand sanitizer before coming into contact with you. And don't be afraid to speak up to staff about your diabetes care.

28 Managing Diabetes in the Hospital: Testing

The stress of illness or injury can make blood sugar levels run high in the hospital, so it's important to keep testing. And since hospital staff may not test as frequently as you'd like, or be as familiar with diabetes care as you are, it's best to be your own advocate. Call the hospital before admission and ask if you will be able to test your own blood sugar while you are an inpatient. If the answer is no, ask to speak with the patient liaison. You can also ask your physician to write orders allowing you to test in the hospital.

29 Managing Diabetes in the Hospital: Meals

Hospital food can contain hidden carbs, even if you ask for a "diabetes-friendly diet." If carbohydrate counts of foods aren't provided on the menu or food labels, ask the dietary staff to provide them so you can avoid any unpleasant surprises.

30 Using D Checklists

A big part of diabetes management is organization. Use checklists as a tool to keep diabetes care tasks from falling through the cracks. You can create master checklists for supplies, for snacks, for meal planning, and for doctor's appointments. Or you can keep a running "To Do" checklist of diabetes-related purchases or tasks you need to complete. Once you find a method that works for you, stick with it.

31 The Diabetes/Colon Cancer Connection

March is Colon Cancer Awareness month. People with type 2 diabetes are at a higher risk for developing colorectal cancer, and those that do develop it face a higher mortality rate. Early detection is critical to beating colorectal cancer. If you are age 50 or older and have not yet had a colonoscopy, ask your doctor about screening today.

April

April is a month of renewed energy and purpose for many as the weather warms up and the world gets greener. Flowers are blooming and vegetable gardens soon will be sprouting. As you "learn something new every day" this month, remember that practicing these healthy lifestyle tips will help them become habits.

▉1 Make the Most of Medical Deductions

Tax day is coming (4/15). The cost of virtually all of your diabetes care and treatment is typically tax deductible. Beyond doctor's visits and prescription drugs, that also includes blood sugar testing supplies and any expenses of a weight-loss program recommended by your doctor. Make sure you keep and track all of these receipts to get the largest medical deduction possible.

▉2 Start Walking

Walking is a cheap and effective way to stay in shape and keep blood sugar in control. Just make sure you invest in three things: (1) a good pair of walking shoes; (2) a small pack to carry essential diabetes supplies in; and (3) a way to track your progress. That can be a high tech activity tracker or as simple as tracking the distance you walk on a map.

▉3 Who Should NOT Drink

While moderate alcohol consumption is fine for most people with diabetes, there are a few exceptions. If you have diabetic neuropathy, kidney disease, or high blood pressure, alcohol can worsen these conditions. When in doubt, ask your doctor.

▉4 Eggs-Cellent Snacks

If you celebrate Easter and have kids or grandkids, you may have an abundance of hard-boiled eggs around this month. A hard-boiled egg is a great source of protein, healthy fats, and vitamins A and D. At just 80 calories and zero carbohydrates, it's a perfect diabetes-friendly snack food.

▉5 Beware of "Low Fat" Labels

Always read the nutrition label on "low fat" versions of packaged food products. When fat is taken out of a food, it is often replaced with high-carb ingredients to add texture. Remember to assess the "Total Carbs" listed on the label before you buy, and compare it to the "regular" full-fat version of the food.

6 April 6 is Fresh Tomato Day

Tomatoes are packed full of disease-fighting antioxidants and are high in Vitamin C and low in calories and carbohydrates. If fresh tomatoes are costly or not yet in season where you live, opt for canned. Canned tomatoes actually contain more cancer-fighting lycopene than fresh ones, making them an excellent nutritional choice for everyone. Just avoid sauces with added sugars that can add unneeded carbs.

7 Healthier Soul Food: Proteins

Soul food is an African American cuisine with a Southern influence. Many traditional soul food recipes are packed with fat, salt, carbs, and calories. But there are ways to make them healthier without sacrificing taste. Bake or roast your favorite chicken recipe instead of frying it. Use hot sauce instead of barbecue sauce to save on calories and carbohydrates. Try some fresh fish seasoned with herbs and spices.

8 Healthier Soul Foods: Sides

Drop the bacon fat, lard, and salt from your side dish recipes. Bake sweet potatoes in their skin. Nutrient-dense collard greens, okra, and black-eyed peas have great natural flavors that you can enhance with herbs and spices. Most cornbread is high in calories and carbohydrates, but you can still have a small piece occasionally if you add in the healthy veggies and keep your overall carbs in check.

9 April Showers and Your Feet

If you are going to spend any length of time outdoors in wet weather, make sure your feet are ready. Invest in waterproof boots and seamless socks that wick moisture away from the skin. If your feet do get wet, dry thoroughly between your toes and check feet carefully for any blisters or abrasions.

Small foot problems can turn into big issues if you don't catch them early.

10 Smart Snacking

Snacks are essential to keeping your blood sugar on a steady course. Since carbs raise blood sugar, spreading them out in small doses throughout the day just makes good sense. So try small midmorning, midafternoon, and bedtime snacks; you may need to experiment with timing and foods. As a rule of thumb, snacks should have about 15 grams of carbohydrates each.

11 Sizing Up Your Dinnerware

Did you know that putting your meals into oversized dishes can actually cause you to overeat? Research has shown that people who use oversized dinnerware eat larger portions and consume more calories during a meal. Plates should be no bigger than 9 inches across. Use small, shallow bowls, and replace short, wide glasses with tall, narrow ones.

12 Gear Up Right

Protect your feet with the right shoes for exercise. Go to a reputable shoe store that specializes in athletic footwear (ask your podiatrist for a referral). Let the clerk know what type of exercise you'll be doing in the shoes so she can make a proper recommendation. If you have foot problems, you may need custom fitted orthotics for your shoes—again, ask your podiatrist for a referral to someone who can custom fit your feet.

13 Counting Casserole Carbs

Here's how to calculate the number of carbohydrates in your favorite casserole recipe. First, look up each ingredient and write down the amount of carbs in each one based on the amount required for the recipe. Add all ingredient carbohydrates together. Then divide this amount by the number of servings that the recipe makes. The result is your "per serving" carb amount.

14 Adding Weight to Your Workout

Unlike aerobic exercise that works your heart and lungs, resistance training works your muscles. Both are important to good diabetes health. Studies show that resistance training improves insulin sensitivity. Try this type of exercise two to three times each week and see what it does for your blood sugar control. If you don't like the gym, buy an inexpensive pair of resistance bands for home training.

15 Eat a Rainbow

Filling half your plate with nonstarchy vegetables at lunch and dinner is a good practice to make sure you are getting enough fiber, vitamins, and minerals. Include a "rainbow" of colors (red, orange, green, purple) in your veggie choices to ensure you are getting a full spectrum of important disease fighting antioxidants and phytochemicals.

16 Fabulous Fungi

April 16th is the Day of the Mushroom. Mushrooms are low in calories and high in fiber, and certain species—including oyster, maitake, and mukitake—may help to improve glycemic control and insulin sensitivity. Add some to a salad, stir-fry, or another favorite dish today.

17 Logging Blood Sugars

Writing down your blood sugar testing numbers, or storing them in an app or computer program, is an important part of diabetes management. A written record helps you detect patterns, and it also makes it easier to share your progress with your doctor.

18 Fruits in Season: Pineapple

Aloha! April is prime time to enjoy Hawaiian pineapple. Pineapple is high in natural sugars, so enjoy it as an occasional treat rather than a daily indulgence. One cup of diced pineapple contains 20 grams of carbohydrates, but it's also packed with health benefits. Pineapple is an excellent source of vitamin C and contains an enzyme called bromelain that helps with the digestion of protein. Bromelain has anti-inflammatory, anticlotting, and anticancer properties.

19 Garlic Day

Vampires beware. April 19th is Garlic Day. And that's good news for you if you have diabetes. Animal studies show garlic (*Allium sativum*) may actually improve insulin resistance. It is in no way a substitute for the medication you already take, but it does make it a good idea to add a healthy dose of garlic to your favorite low-carb dish.

20 Know Your Zeitgeibers

A zeitgeiber is an environmental cue that helps regulate circadian rhythms and sleep. Bright light is a major zeitgeiber. It triggers chemical messengers that act on the brain and wake us or make us tired. Keeping the sleep environment as dark as possible, and avoiding "screen light" from phones, tablets, and computers, is critical to getting good sleep, and sleeping well is an important part of maintaining good blood sugar control.

21 Do You Need a Pedorthist?

A pedorthist is a person trained in the design, fabrication, and fit of orthotics—shoe inserts that are custom fit to your feet. If you have a history of foot ulcers or conditions that alter the shape of your foot (e.g., Charcot foot), you should ask your podiatrist about a referral to a pedorthist. Health insurance often covers the cost.

22 Smart Sharps Disposal

Today is Earth Day. Diabetes generates a lot of unavoidable medical waste. We can minimize the impact it has on the environment by disposing of it properly. Needles can be dangerous to the earth and to waste handlers when they are thrown out with the regular trash. Your waste hauler or public works department can tell you the procedure for proper disposal in your area. Many pharmacies also have needle disposal programs.

23 Could It Be Gastroparesis?

Gastroparesis is a form of nerve damage to the digestive system that can occur in people with diabetes. When nerves in the stomach and gastrointestinal tract aren't working properly, digestion slows, resulting in symptoms such as nausea, constipation, erratic blood sugar levels, and bloating. If you are experiencing any of these, talk to your doctor. Treatment options are available.

24 The Yard-Workout

Exercise doesn't have to involve a gym membership or special machines or classes. Just working in your yard to keep up the landscaping can have health benefits. The following activities all burn about 150 calories: gardening for 30 to 45 minutes; raking leaves for 30 minutes; mowing the lawn for 30 minutes; and shoveling snow for 15 minutes.

25 The Fatigue-Hunger Connection

Ever notice yourself getting hungry when you haven't had enough sleep? There's a biological reason for that. When we don't sleep enough our levels of leptin (the "all full" hormone) decrease, and ghrelin (the hunger hormone) increase, creating a recipe for weight gain. If you are sleep deprived, eating small, healthy meals on a regular schedule may help combat hunger.

26 Mock Mac and Cheese

Miss your high-carb mac and cheese? Try this surprising substitute. Steam a whole head of cauliflower and transfer it to a casserole or soufflé dish. Mix one tablespoon of mayo and one teaspoon Dijon mustard, spread the mixture on the head of cauliflower, then dot with one to two tablespoons of butter. Sprinkle with a half cup of Parmesan cheese and bake at 350°F for 15 minutes or until golden brown, then scoop and serve.

27 Handling Head Pain

Headache can be a symptom of either a high or low blood sugar level. If a headache hits you out of nowhere, check your blood sugar. Headache is also a common side effect of many diabetes drugs. If you have chronic head pain, talk to your doctor. He may be able to adjust your medication to resolve the headaches, or refer you to a neurologist or headache specialist if it isn't diabetes related.

28 Tex-Mex Remix

Here's how to lower the carb content of your favorite Southwestern fare. Use corn or whole wheat tortillas instead of regular tortillas, and choose fresh seafood, lean poultry, and dried beans as your protein source for tacos or enchiladas. Instead of buying canned refried beans, drain and rinse whole black beans or pinto beans and put them in the food processor with your favorite spices. Along with fresh salsa, use plain Greek yogurt instead of sour cream as a topping.

29 Heat Things Up With Salsa Dancing

Salsa dancing works a variety of the muscles in your body, mostly around your hips, legs, and hard-to-tone arms. It won't hurt your knees like running, and you can burn a bunch of calories while you enjoy the beat of the invigorating Latin music. Salsa dancing can improve your balance, flexibility, posture, and coordination, and give you energy to boot! Check your local dance studio or gym for classes, or find a "how-to" video.

30 Slow Down on Sugar Alcohols

Sugar alcohols, or polyols, are substances that are added to foods and drinks to sweeten without added calories and carbohydrates. Common sugar alcohols include sorbitol, mannitol, xylitol, and others. They are found in many foods labeled "sugar free." When you see sugar alcohol listed on the food label, make sure you eat the food in moderation. In large amounts, sugar alcohols can have a laxative affect.

May

Ladies, take time to celebrate your health this May during National Women's Health Week, which starts on Mother's Day each year. This month's tips help you take care of yourself and your family (and there's plenty for the men, too).

1. Spring Clean Your Diet

Spring is a great time to clean out your closets and clean up your eating plan. Pave a path to clean eating by adding in fresh vegetables for snacks. Cut up a cucumber or bite into a red pepper instead of reaching for a cookie or granola bar. You'll reap the benefits of adding in a low-calorie, high-fiber snack and reduce your intake of processed food at the same time.

2. Spring Clean Your Supplies

Update your diabetes supplies as part of your spring cleaning ritual. Make sure your testing supplies (including your blood sugar meter and related equipment) are in optimal condition with fresh batteries. Get rid of items that are expired or that you no longer use. Check with local government agencies to find out how to dispose of expired or unwanted medications or pills.

3. Get Your Diabetes in the Bag

There are a variety of stylish diabetes supply organizers out there to choose from. Buy something fun and functional and you'll be less likely to forget it at home. Myabetic, aDorn, and Sugar Medical are just a few of the companies that specialize in supply bags for both women and men.

4. May Is Mediterranean Diet Month

The Mediterranean diet is a heart-healthy eating plan that may help you lose weight and gain control over your blood sugar levels. It is high in olive oil, vegetables, fruits, grains, beans, and fish. There is good research that shows this type of an eating plan may be helpful for its protective effects again cardiovascular disease, stroke, some cancers, and reducing the risk for developing type 2 diabetes.

5. Testing Tip: Multiple Meters

Easy access to a glucose meter will allow you to test as often as needed so you can improve your daily diabetes management. Keep several in the places you spend the most time (e.g., work, home, and school). Never try to guess your blood sugar, especially if you are feeling symptoms of a high or low; always test to be sure.

6. Today Is National "No Diet Day"

Many people go on a "diet" to lose weight at some time during their lives. But research now tells us that dramatically restricting calories actually triggers hormonal changes that will eventually cause weight *gain*. Instead of "dieting," start to make small but permanent life changes. Have a healthy breakfast and prepare your lunch and snacks for the day. You'll soon be on your way to becoming more fit and healthy.

7. Don't Get Freezer Burned

Although foods with freezer burn are safe to eat, they look unappetizing and can taste dry and tough. To prevent getting burned, store your food in proper size freezer containers with a moisture-vapor barrier. If you use freezer bags, push as much air out of them as you can before closing. For long-term freezer storage, vacuum sealers are best because they remove all of the air from the container.

8. Battling Anxiety

Anxiety is a common issue for people who have diabetes. In addition to worrying about family and work issues, you may also be anxious about managing your blood sugars, food, and medications on a daily basis. You're not alone! Try taking a leisurely walk, keeping a journal, or practicing deep breathing exercises. You may need to speak with a licensed therapist, who may recommend antianxiety medication. Ask your doctor for help.

9. Picking Perfect Produce

When possible, buy fruits and vegetables that are in season. Your produce will be fresher, taste better, and you will spend less money at the same time. Artichokes, asparagus, broccoli, collards, and spinach are all in season during the month of May.

10 Getting Your Game On

Tapping into your inner athlete is a great way to help to control your blood sugar levels. You are also more likely to stick with exercise you enjoy, so if you love the camaraderie of softball or the competitive challenge of tennis, channel that passion into a healthy routine. Even on days you don't have a game, you can get some heart pumping practice in.

11 Pregnancy and Diabetes

Pregnancy is a remarkable journey, but it can be especially challenging when you have diabetes. It's very important to speak to your endocrinologist and OB-GYN about your blood sugar levels and health *before* you become pregnant. Working with a health care team that understands you and your diabetes will help keep you and your baby healthy during your pregnancy.

12 Safely Storing Fruits and Veggies

Store produce properly so it doesn't spoil or lose flavor before you are ready to eat it. Most fruits and veggies should not be cleaned until you are ready to eat them. Wash tough-skinned produce such as melons, avocado, and squash before cutting them. Once you cut up honeydew and cantaloupe, they should be refrigerated. Keep your tomatoes and bananas on the counter, and store potatoes in a cool dark place in your pantry.

13 Menopause and Blood Sugar

During menopause, the hormones estrogen and progesterone affect how your body responds to insulin. You may notice that your blood sugars fluctuate more. You may also experience weight gain, which can influence the amount of medications you require. Keep track of your blood sugar more often during the day, and test occasionally at night, too. If you keep a detailed journal of your patterns and share it with your endocrinologist, he or she may be able to help you make adjustments.

14 Living Well After Menopause

If you are suffering from hot flashes, vaginal dryness, sleep problems, and anxiety due to menopause, there are a number of treatments that are available, but you must discuss these issues openly with your health care provider. You should also ask your doctor and certified diabetes educator about ways to adjust your current eating plan and exercise program to help you manage your menopausal symptoms and blood sugars.

15 Get Your Annual Eye Exam

People with diabetes should get a dilated eye exam every year. You may not feel any pain or visual blurring during the early stages of diabetic retinopathy, but if retinopathy is spotted in its early stages on an annual eye exam, excellent treatments are available. Simply put, the earlier eye disease is found, the easier it is to treat. Make your annual eye appointment today!

16 Seeing Clearly

Fluctuating blood sugars can cause changes in vision. It's important to get your blood sugars under reasonable control before seeing your eye doctor and getting an updated prescription and a new pair of glasses. However, once you know that your blood sugars are in an acceptable range, make sure to see your eye doctor. Your vision may have changed and a new pair of glasses may be in order.

17 Signs You Should Get to the Eye Doctor

If you are experiencing changes in your vision (blurriness, floaters, dark spots, or flashing lights) or eye pain, call your eye doctor right away. Early detection of eye diseases like macular degeneration or glaucoma is important, so don't wait for your annual eye exam if you have any of these warning signs.

18 Fruits in Season: Apricots

Apricots are a delicious sweet treat that are in season during the month of May. Select an apricot that is an orange or yellow-orange color, firm to the touch, and looks nice and plump. If the apricots are not quite ripe when you buy them, store them in a brown paper bag for two to three days. If your apricot is ripe, "twist it" gently. It will quickly break in half for your eating enjoyment.

19 Gesundheit!

Although springtime allergies may not directly affect your blood sugar levels, you need to be careful when selecting a remedy for your sneezing and itching. Many antihistamines can cause drowsiness, so be sure not to miss your diabetes medications or meals if your sleep habits are affected by them. Talk to your pharmacist about the possible effects these over-the-counter medications may have on your blood sugar levels.

20 Flex Your Green Thumb

There is nothing more delicious than a ripe tomato picked directly off the vine in your very own garden. Start with a small garden. You will need good soil, plenty of water, and a good amount of direct sunshine. Divide a bed into square-foot sections, and make sure you read the specific planting directions of each vegetable. Try planting tomatoes, eggplants, and peppers, which will grow well with just a little TLC.

21 Choosing Heart Smart Oils

Canola, olive, and sunflower are just a few cooking oils that are high in heart-healthy unsaturated fat, and taste good to boot. Although these oils have the same amount of calories as unhealthy fats, they have a number of different health benefits. Try them on your salads and in your favorite recipes.

22 Know Your Cycle

Monitor your blood sugars carefully before, during, and directly after your period, as hormonal changes during your cycle influence your diabetes control. Tracking any changes in your blood sugar levels will help you recognize trends for next month and plan for your needed adjustments to food, insulin, or medications. Regular exercise can be very effective in managing blood sugar levels in women with type 2 diabetes who may be insulin resistant.

23 Great Grain Swaps

Whole grains are a great source of fiber, selenium, potassium, and magnesium, and people who eat whole grains are at lower risk to develop heart disease and certain cancers. So toss out your dry Italian bread crumbs and use rolled oats instead. Try replacing white rice with bulgur, barley, or kasha. If you have celiac disease, opt for gluten-free grains such as buckwheat, corn, and wild rice.

24 Diagnosing Celiac Disease

People with type 1 diabetes are at higher risk for developing celiac disease. If you are going to get tested, it's important that you not yet cut gluten completely out of your diet. Dropping gluten can reduce levels of the antibodies that the test looks for in your blood, producing a false negative. If you have already gone gluten free but need to be tested for celiac, your doctor may request that you add gluten back into your diet for a specified period of time before taking the test.

25 Going Gluten Free for Life

If you are diagnosed with celiac disease, then you should meet with a registered dietitian nutritionist to learn about the principles of a gluten-free diet. A gluten-free menu would exclude wheat, rye, barley, malt, and several other grains. Remember that fresh meats, fish, fruits, and vegetables are all gluten free. So are grains such as buckwheat and quinoa.

26 Hidden Glutens

If you have celiac disease, you already know to avoid breads, cereals, and crackers, which contain gluten. But gluten can be hidden in places you never thought of looking. Check your pantry for packaged products containing soy sauce, malt, or other gluten-containing ingredients. If you plan on dining out, do some research in advance to be sure the restaurant offers gluten-free dishes.

27 It's UV Awareness Month

If you spend time outdoors, it's important to protect yourself from the sun's ultraviolet (UV) rays. Always use a sunscreen with a sun protection factor (SPF) of 30 or higher. Take a break from the sun (especially between the hours of 10 a.m. to 4 p.m.), and find a shady spot to relax for a while. Make sure you wear a hat at the beach or pool, and sunglasses to protect your eyes and the area around them.

28 National Senior Health and Fitness Day

Exercise improves your cardiovascular and bone health along with lowering your blood sugar levels. But you have to be careful not to overdo it, especially if you have joint problems or arthritis. Get guidance from your doctor on what a safe level of activity is for you. And always make sure to warm up before you start your workout.

29 The Art of Packing

Plan your packing. Make a list of all of the clothes, essential toiletries, and diabetes supplies that you will need for your trip. That way you'll never forget anything that you need and you can purchase last minute items prior to your trip (saving you time, money, and aggravation). Have a lot of clothes to bring? Roll, rather than fold. You'll be able to put a lot more in your suitcase.

30 Traveling with Diabetes

Always bring at least twice the amount of diabetes supplies and medications that you need. If your return trip is delayed, you'll have everything you need with you. And whether you're traveling by land, air, or water, always keep testing supplies, insulin, medications, and other diabetes essentials where they can be easily accessed.

31 It's World No Tobacco Day

Quitting smoking is the single most important thing you can do for your health. But nicotine withdrawal can be very tough. You may feel ill, depressed, and irritable the first few days without a cigarette. Emotional support from family and friends is extremely important when you are trying to quit smoking. You may want to consider behavior therapy in combination with nicotine replacement.

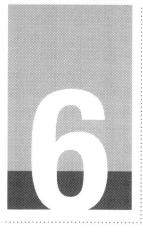

June

May was for the ladies, and June is for the guys. It's Men's Health Month and time to focus on the unique needs of men with diabetes. You'll also find plenty of great nutrition and treatment tips for everyone.

1. Low T and Diabetes

Many men with type 2 diabetes also have low testosterone levels, which are linked to insulin resistance and reduced insulin sensitivity. If you are overweight, weight loss will help control both your diabetes and your testosterone levels. Continue to eat a heart-healthy diet and exercise every day. Testosterone replacement therapy may also be an option. Discuss your options with your doctor.

2. Talking to Your Doctor: What Men Should Know

Studies show us that men are less likely to see a doctor for emerging health issues than women are. But the simple fact is that you just can't do this when you have diabetes. Easy to treat issues can turn into serious, chronic problems. So don't try to "do it yourself" when you have an injury or illness. Let your doctor be your partner in health care.

3. Stay on Your Toes with Foot Care

If your feet or legs have nerve damage, even a small cut can lead to serious problems. Inspect your feet daily and speak to your doctor if you have cuts or breaks in the skin or an ingrown toenail. Let them know if your foot changes color or becomes extremely sensitive or painful. If you can't see the bottom of your feet, use a mirror. Do it at the same time each day so you don't forget.

4. Dressing for Success

Salad dressings can make an otherwise mundane salad come to life. But many dressings have hidden carbohydrates. Try this homemade low-carb salad dressing. Start with ¾ of a cup of red wine or balsamic vinegar and ¼ cup of olive oil. Squeeze in some fresh lemon, a dash of oregano, minced garlic, and spicy brown mustard to taste. Whisk it all together and voila! You've put your own personal stamp on your salad.

5 Meditating for Stress Relief

Try this meditation exercise to de-stress. Sit in a comfortable position and close your eyes. Breathe in deeply from your diaphragm and breathe out slowly from your nose. Repeat three to five times while you concentrate on your breathing. When you breathe in, think the words "I am," and as you exhale, think the words "in peace." You'll soon start to feel a little more centered and calm.

6 Veggies in Season: Green Beans

Green beans are rich in thiamine, riboflavin, and niacin. One cup of fresh green beans provides only 31 calories, 7 grams of carbohydrates, 3 grams of fiber, and 2 grams of protein. Dip raw green beans in fresh salsa for a tasty snack, or steam them, drizzle with olive oil, and top with sliced almonds.

7 How to Choose Yogurt

Many yogurts contain added sugars. Low-fat plain Greek yogurt may be your best choice, as it's high in protein and lower in carbohydrates. Yogurt can also be a good source of probiotics, the good bacteria that help to keep your digestive tract working properly. As always, read the labels, and choose yogurts with *Lactobacillus acidophilus*, *Lactobacillus casei*, *Bifidobacterium bifidum*, or *Bifidobacterium longum*.

8 Understanding the Glycemic Index

You can use the glycemic index (GI) in conjunction with carb counting to help control your blood sugars. The GI is a numerical value from 0 to 100 that indicates how a carbohydrate-containing food will affect your blood sugar level. Low GI foods (≤55) digest slowly and cause a slower rise in blood sugar levels than high GI foods. There are websites and apps available that list the GI of various foods.

9 GI: Form and Cooking Matter

The more a food is processed, the higher its glycemic index. For example, orange juice has a higher GI than a whole orange.

Cooking method also matters; the GI of raw carrots is lower than the GI of cooked carrots. If you are using GI as a tool to help plan meals, make sure you are finding the right form of your food on GI lists.

10 It's National Herbs and Spices Day

Add flavor to your recipes with onion, garlic, ginger, and oregano. Or spice things up with chili powder, tarragon, and red pepper flakes to give some bite to meals without the added sodium. The following spices may even improve insulin sensitivity: cinnamon, curry, basil, garlic, nutmeg, ginger, cumin, and fenugreek.

11 Visiting the Podiatrist

Take a step toward better diabetes management and make your annual appointment with a podiatrist. Your podiatrist can safely remove calluses and cut your toenails, so you don't risk injury or infection. During your visit, make sure to review proper daily foot care techniques and discuss footwear, especially if you are having any issues with your feet.

12 The Power of Peer Support

Sometimes people with diabetes feel alone and isolated. Peer support can help, but men may be less likely to seek out this resource. Do yourself a favor and commit to one support group meeting to test the waters. You may find that talking to other people who have similar experiences with the daily management of diabetes can be very empowering.

13 Finding a Good Fit

When trying to find the right "support group fit" for your needs, talk to the person running the group. Don't be shy! Ask questions to make sure you can address your specific needs. Like shoe shopping, you may find you have to "try on" a few groups before you discover one that fits comfortably.

14 | Bone and Joint Health

Keeping your bones strong is essential if you have diabetes. Exercise helps to keep diabetes under better control and maintains strong bones at the same time. Make sure you include plenty of calcium, vitamin D, and vitamin K in your diet to keep your bones healthy. If you are concerned about your bone health, ask your doctor about a bone density test to determine if you are at risk for osteoporosis.

15 | ED and Diabetes

Erectile dysfunction (ED) is common in men who have diabetes. The problem may be related to poor blood sugar control, which damages nerves and blood vessels. It could also be linked to high blood pressure or coronary artery disease. Be open with your doctor if you are having trouble getting or sustaining an erection. There are many treatment options today to treat ED, but you have to talk about it first.

16 | "Before and After" Testing

Testing your blood sugar before and after meals, before and after exercise, or even before or after sleeping can help you detect patterns of highs or lows and troubleshoot problems. Pick a pair of tests to take and compare the results over the course of the week. It's also a good way to become more aware of changes in your blood sugar levels throughout the week, or at least get you to start testing more often!

17 | Get Regular Checkups

Make sure that you get an annual checkup with your health care provider. Physicals, including EKG's, full blood panels, blood pressure checks, and general health screenings, can help prevent more serious health issues. It's important to have your weight and vital signs checked as well, and discuss any significant changes or issues that may be of concern.

18 Eat Slowly

It takes about 15 to 20 minutes for our hormonal and brain signals to let us know if we have satiated our hunger. If you do find yourself cleaning your plate quickly, let some time pass before going back for seconds so your brain can catch up with your body.

19 Men, Diabetes, and Depression

Diabetes doubles the risk of depression. Men are less likely to express the "typical" symptoms of depression such as crying and sadness, but they may become outwardly irritable or angry. Depression can prevent you from taking care of yourself and may eventually affect your blood sugars, so it's important to talk to your doctor and get help.

20 Spike Stopping Vinegar

Adding vinegar to your diet may help to improve blood sugar levels and glycemic control if you have type 2 diabetes. The acetic acid found in vinegar may combat the action of certain enzymes, causing some sugars and starches to temporarily pass through the intestines without being digested. As a result, the impact on your blood sugar is lowered. Try drizzling vinegar and olive oil over your veggies and salads.

21 Metformin and Medical Tests

If you take metformin, one of the most common oral diabetes drugs, be careful when scheduling radiology tests. The contrast medium used in CT scans and some other radiological procedures reacts with metformin and can hurt your kidneys. You may need to discontinue the metformin for a short time, or your doctor may suggest a different procedure.

22 Is CGM Right for You?

A continuous glucose monitor (CGM) is a way to measure glucose levels in real-time throughout the day and overnight. It doesn't completely replace finger stick testing, but it does show trends and patterns in blood sugar levels that can help you prevent hypo- and hyperglycemia. Ask your doctor if they can prescribe a three- to seven-day trial session so you can see what it's like to use a CGM.

23 Avoid Energy Drinks

So-called "energy drinks" usually contain more than twice as much caffeine than a regular cup of coffee or cola, and a lot of sugar. Studies show that drinking too many energy drinks may increase blood pressure and heart rate, and may be dangerous for people with diabetes and high blood pressure. Try to avoid these drinks, but if you must have one occasionally, make it the sugar-free type.

24 Sweeping Time

Have trouble managing your time in the morning to fit in all the diabetes self-care tasks you need to? Replace your digital clock with an "old school" analog one. Seeing the physical sweep of time is often a more powerful motivator than seeing electronic numbers on a screen. Analog clocks are fairly inexpensive, so try putting one in the bathroom, one in the kitchen, and one in your bedroom.

25 Your Diabetes Guide

A certified diabetes educator (CDE) can help you gain the knowledge and skills that you need to care for your diabetes. Whether you are newly diagnosed, need a "refresher" course, or are simply overwhelmed with your management after so many years of dealing with this disease, a CDE can help guide you toward better control.

26 Smart Snacking with Salsa

Make fresh salsa, and use it as a dip for cut up veggies. Dice fresh onions, tomatoes, a jalapeno pepper, and cilantro, place in a bowl and add olive oil, minced garlic, and a dash of cumin. If you can't live without tortilla chips, make sure you count out one serving into a dish. It's too easy to overeat out of the chip bag.

27 To Refrigerate or Not to Refrigerate

Have you ever wondered why some of your fruits and vegetables spoil before you've had a chance to enjoy them? It may be how you are storing them. Keep your artichokes, asparagus, berries, broccoli, and carrots in the refrigerator. Store apples, avocados, and bananas at room temperature. Make sure that you store your fruits and vegetables separately in the refrigerator, as some vegetables produce ethylene gas that promotes the ripening process.

28 Fats to Stay Away From

There have been recent studies that bring into question whether saturated fat is actually as bad for heart health as once thought. The jury is still out as research in this area is still evolving. What we do know for certain is that trans fat can hurt your cardiovascular system. It raises LDL (low density lipoprotein, or "bad" cholesterol), and increases the risk of heart disease and stroke. Choose foods with "0g trans fat" listed on the nutrition label.

29 The 15–15 Rule

If your blood sugar is below 70 mg/dL (hypoglycemia), use the 15–15 rule. Take 15 grams of carbohydrates and recheck your blood sugar in 15 minutes. If your blood sugar is still low, take another 15 grams of carbohydrates and retest again in 15 minutes. Some examples of 15 grams of carbohydrates are three to four glucose tablets (check the package for glucose amount), 15 grams of glucose gel, 4 ounces of fruit juice, or 1 tablespoon of sugar.

30 Crossing Time Zones

You may need to change your insulin and medication schedule when you travel between time zones. If you travel east, you will have a shorter day, so you may need less insulin. If you travel west, you will have a longer day and more insulin may be required. If the time difference is less than three hours, you should be able to stick to your normal regimen. Discuss your travel schedule with your doctor at least six weeks before your trip to go over any adjustments.

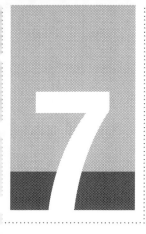

July

Summer is in full swing and so is sun, fun, and fireworks. This month we share advice on how to safely manage the blood sugar challenges of the season.

1 Hot Weather and Supply Safety

Hot and humid weather can have an effect on your diabetes supplies. Never leave an insulin pump, blood sugar meter, test strips, or medication in a hot car. If you are out in the heat, keep all of your supplies out of direct sunlight and in an insulated bag to ensure they stay safe.

2 Heat and Blood Sugar

Make a few smart adjustments to control your blood sugar during the dog days of summer. Avoid dehydration by drinking plenty of water, especially if you are exercising or doing yard work outdoors. If you become dehydrated, your blood sugar may rise. Don't confuse heat related issues (such as light-headedness and confusion) with low blood sugar. Make sure you test your blood sugars often.

3 Smart Summer Footwear

Although it may be tempting to run around barefoot over the summer, don't. If you cut your foot on something sharp (indoors or outside), you can get an infection. Avoid flip-flops and sandals, which leave your feet exposed and could cause blisters or sores. Make sure to wear shoes that protect the whole foot, are comfortable, and fit well, as your feet may swell during the summer heat.

4 Independence Day Food and Fun

July 4th is a day of fun, friends, family, and food! Fill up on some fresh veggies dipped in salsa or hummus, and keep your distance from chips and high-calorie/high-carb dips. Enjoy a burger or hot dog if you'd like, but make sure you use a small plate and limit the macaroni and potato salad. Have a refreshing bowl of blueberries and strawberries topped with Greek yogurt for a patriotic dessert.

5 Low-Carb Summer Fruits

Summer is a great time to enjoy fresh, juicy fruits. Try blueberries, strawberries, blackberries, and raspberries for a luscious summertime snack. Indulge in a slice of watermelon, or savor an apricot, plum, or kiwi. Fruits are a great source of antioxidants, vitamins, minerals, and fiber, and should be part of your healthy meal plan. Just make sure to monitor your portion sizes.

6 Veggies in Season: Cucumbers

Cucumbers are cool and refreshing, and half a cup of sliced cucumber has only 8 calories! They are also low in saturated fat and sodium, and a good source of vitamin A, magnesium (which can help lower your blood sugar), phosphorus, manganese, vitamin C, vitamin K, and potassium. Slice up a cuke on your salad, or hollow out half a cucumber and fill it with sandwich stuffings for a lower-carb alternative to bread.

7 Picnic Prep Safety

Celebrate a lovely summer day with a picnic. Don't forget a food thermometer, ice for your cooler, storage containers, paper towels, trash bags, and your diabetes supplies. Keep your meat cold until it's time to grill. Use the meat thermometer to check the internal temperature and make sure your meat or chicken is safe to eat. Never use the same plate or utensils for the raw meat and your cooked food.

8 Packing Up Your Picnic

Use a well-insulated cooler or insulated bags with ice packs to pack up your leftovers. Keep any leftover raw meat in a separate cooler or well-sealed separate container to avoid contaminating other food. If the temperature is over 80°F outside, don't bring home leftovers that have been outdoors for more than one hour. Unpack as you arrive home, and refrigerate leftovers immediately.

9 Refrigerating Insulin

If you keep your insulin in the refrigerator, make sure you can clearly see the expiration date. The expiration date will usually be one year from when you purchased it, but make sure to always check the box to make sure. Once the bottle is opened, make sure to use it within one month (write the date opened on the label). Never store your insulin in the freezer or in direct sunlight.

10 How to Stay Hydrated

Use a reusable water bottle that you can carry with you wherever you go. Sip your water throughout the day, and take a few extra gulps before meals. Use an app that tracks water intake and reminds you to drink more, or set alarms on your smartphone to remind you to drink up. Add sliced lemon, lime, cucumber, or a bit of mint to your water to make it more interesting without adding carbs or calories.

11 How Often Should You See Your Diabetes Doctor?

You should see your endocrinologist or diabetes doctor at least twice a year. If you are taking insulin or having diabetes-related issues, you may need to increase this to every three months. In addition to these diabetes visits, you should make regular appointments with your certified diabetes educator (CDE), podiatrist, eye doctor, dentist, and other members of your health care team.

12 Bug Bites

Bug bites are an unavoidable part of summer. Place an ice pack on the sting or bite for 15 to 20 minutes once an hour for a few hours. Do not fall asleep with ice on your skin, and elevate the area to bring down the swelling. Check with your doctor before you use over-the-counter medicine to relieve pain or itching. If you develop fever, hives, or significant swelling after a bug bite, contact your doctor immediately.

13 Sunburn Safety

Sunburn can cause a rise in blood sugar levels. And if you develop a serious sunburn with blisters, you risk infection. Of course, shade, sunscreen, a hat, and protective clothing are your first defense to reduce sun overexposure. But if you do get burnt, try using aloe, which can be very soothing. And if your skin blisters, see your doctor for appropriate treatment.

14 Words to Know: Basal vs. Bolus

Basal and bolus refer to insulin doses. Basal insulin is insulin that works slowly and steadily throughout the day. A bolus of insulin is a larger, fast-acting dose of insulin given at mealtime to compensate for the upcoming blood sugar rise from carbohydrates. Some insulin types are designed for basal dosing (intermediate- and long-acting) and others for bolusing before meals (fast- or rapid-acting). Your doctor will individualize your insulin therapy for you.

15 Skip the Diet Soda

Recent studies link diet soda with an increased risk of developing type 2 diabetes, metabolic syndrome, and heart disease. More research is needed, but scientists believe that the artificial sweeteners may trick your body into thinking that it wants more carbohydrates, which can ultimately result in weight gain for heavy-duty diet soda drinkers. Although you may not have to cut diet soda out of your life completely, try to drink it in moderation.

16 Be a CGM Detective

Use your continuous glucose monitor (CGM) for more than just catching highs and lows. By being a "CGM detective" you can figure out what snacks and meals are best before and after your workouts, and if you need to increase the amount of carbohydrates you need during exercise. You may also be able to change the timing of your insulin to better match your meals and activity level. Share the data with your doctor and together you can solve mysterious blood sugar bounces.

17 Giving Blood with Diabetes

Many adults with diabetes can donate blood. There are a few prerequisites. Your blood sugar should be in good control, and you should have an adequate hemoglobin level. If you have used bovine (beef) insulin made in the United Kingdom since 1980, you are not allowed to donate blood due to the concern over "mad cow disease."

18 Fruits in Season: Peaches

Peaches are a sweet and juicy fruit, which are commonly available in the clingstone and freestone varieties. A medium peach has about 60 calories and 14 grams of carbohydrates and is rich in vitamins A and C, potassium, and fiber. Pick a peach that is firm or slightly soft and free of bruises.

19 Understanding Net Carbs

The term "net carbs" is not endorsed by the U.S. Food and Drug Administration (FDA). Processed food manufacturers came up with the term, and define net carbs as the total grams of carbohydrates minus the grams of sugar alcohols, fiber, and glycerine. This formula is flawed because sugar alcohols and fiber are partially absorbed by the body and may impact blood sugar. Always pay attention to "total carbohydrate" amounts, and don't be misled by marketing campaigns.

20 Dish Sizes Matter

Ever go to a restaurant and get your entrée on a plate the size of a hubcap? Standard plate sizes have increased from around 9 inches in the 1960s to over 12 inches today. The larger your plate, the more you are likely to eat a bigger portion. It's easy to control this at home, but when you eat out, remember that your eyes may deceive you. One trick is to hang on to the small plate you get for bread and appetizers and transfer a reasonable serving from your entrée plate to it.

21 Efficient Appointment Scheduling

Diabetes means lots of doctor's appointments, which can translate to a lot of time on the telephone. To save yourself time and phone tag headaches, avoid calling first thing in the morning or around lunch, when you are less likely to get through. Ask office staff for the best times of day to reach them. And if your doctor's office has an online portal, take advantage of its appointment request features.

22 The Seven Self-Care Behaviors

CDEs focus on seven main areas of diabetes care: healthy eating, being active, monitoring, taking medication, problem solving, reducing risk, and healthy coping. If you are struggling in any of these areas, it's time to see a diabetes educator. No need to keep battling alone!

23 Tracking Your Every Move

Some people find that fitness trackers can be a huge motivator in getting enough movement each day. You can also pick your level of technological comfort. There's a wide range of products available, from simple step-counting pedometers to more advanced fitness bands that calculate calories burned and track heart rate. Talk to your CDE for a recommendation that fits your lifestyle and budget.

24 Spotting Spoiled Insulin

Always check the expiration date of your insulin before you draw it up. Then take a moment to inspect the bottle. Rapid- and short-acting insulin should be clear, but intermediate-acting insulin should look cloudy. The long-lasting insulins, glargine (Lantus) and detemir (Levemir), should be clear. If your insulin has any crystals or debris in it, or looks cloudy when it should be clear, it could be expired or spoiled. When in doubt, throw it out.

25 A Healthy Chip Swap

Put down the high-carb, high-calorie, high-fat potato chips, and try crispy and flavorful kale chips instead. To make kale chips, wash and dry the kale completely and tear it into bite size pieces. Drizzle a small amount of olive oil on the kale and spread it on a baking sheet. Add a little garlic powder and pepper for more taste. Bake it at 350°F for about 10 minutes or until crispy. Kale cooks quickly, so make sure it doesn't burn.

26 Hot and Sticky

If you sweat in the summer heat, you might notice that the adhesive tape on your pump infusion set or CGM sensor becomes loose. Discuss your skin preparation technique with your doctor. Believe it or not, an antiperspirant spray has a compound that may help the tape stick. Before you put on your next set or sensor, try using a spritz of antiperspirant at the site first.

27 Don't Go Barefoot

Although you might enjoy walking barefoot outside over the warm summer months, always wear something on your feet. If you have diabetes, you are at risk for peripheral neuropathy, and you may not feel breaks in your skin or to the bottom of your feet. If you are at the beach, sand could get into an open wound or into your cracked feet and cause unwanted issues.

28 Perfecting Your Pizza Order

Does pizza send your blood sugar into orbit? The amount and type of pizza you eat can affect your blood sugar in different ways. For example, a lot of added fat from extra cheese and toppings can delay a rise in blood sugar. And thick crust will amp up the carb count. Start small, with one slice of thin crust pizza, and test your blood sugar before and after. It may take a bit of trial and error to figure out your best pizza strategy.

29 Beer and Blood Sugar

Ice cold beer is a mainstay at many summer picnics and gatherings. Remember that beer, like all alcohol, can trigger a low blood sugar episode. Always make sure to check your blood sugar before, during, and after drinking alcohol and before bed. To slow down alcohol absorption, always eat before cracking open a cold one. Try not to drink beer when you exercise, because working out can lower your blood sugar as well.

30 Cool Tips for Insulin

Try using a protective pouch with a small cold gel pack to protect your insulin from the hot temperatures. Cooling wallets can keep insulin, pens, and pumps at a safe temperature, without the need for refrigeration, for up to 48 hours. They are reusable too!

31 A Handful of Heart Health

Did you know that 12 tart cherries have only 59 calories and 14 grams of carbohydrates? Some research indicates that the anti-inflammatory agents and antioxidants in tart cherries may help fight heart disease. This makes them the perfect pick for a seasonal snack.

August

The dog days of summer can make things like outdoor exercise and healthy cooking harder to achieve. Fortunately, there are ways to work around summer's heat and enjoy the sun while keeping your blood sugar under control.

1. Surfs Up

Headed to the beach? Keep a few safety tips in mind. Slather on plenty of sunscreen and consider a sun umbrella for protection; like any injury, sunburn can drive up blood sugar. Even though it's tempting, don't go barefoot—protect your feet with aqua shoes if you are walking in sand or water.

2. Low-Carb Liquids

Water is always a great standby for summer, but it can get boring. Try a water infuser bottle to jazz up your water with citrus fruit, watermelon, or berries. Real lemonade is also a good choice if you are using sweeteners that are low in calories and carbohydrates; lemons are high in vitamin C and their acidity means they have a low glycemic index, so they may be kinder to your blood sugar levels.

3. Exercising Outdoors

Hot weather and activity can make dehydration come on quickly. Drink plenty of water before, during, and after exercise. To ward off heat exhaustion on steamy summer days, plan your exercise for early morning or early evening hours, when the temps are cooler. An air-conditioned gym or a swimming pool are also options for managing workouts during a heat wave.

4. Driving with Diabetes

A low blood sugar while driving could be fatal for you or someone else. Always test before you drive. If your blood sugar is 70 mg/dL or lower, treat the low and don't drive until you are back in a safe range. If you ever start to feel symptoms of a low while driving, pull over immediately to test and treat it (keeping glucose tablets in your glove compartment is always a good idea).

5 Testing When You Travel Abroad

The United States is the only country in the world to use mg/dL as a blood sugar testing result value; the rest of the world uses mmol/L as a measurement. Dividing the mg/dL value by 18 will calculate the mmol/L value for you. For example, 100 mg/dL is 5.6 mmol/L. So if you visit a doctor or need to purchase a meter abroad for any reason, don't be shocked by the difference in numbers.

6 Veggies in Season: Edamame

Edamame, or green soybeans, are the only vegetable that contains all nine essential amino acids, making them a "complete protein." They make a tasty snack when boiled or baked and sprinkled with your favorite seasoning (eat them shelled or right out of the pod). You can also cook them up in a stir-fry, toss them in a salad, or add them to soup and casseroles. A ½ cup serving has 110 calories, 10 grams of carbohydrates, and 1 gram of fiber.

7 Probiotics and Diabetes

Probiotics are "good bacteria" that thrive in the gut and aid in digestion. They can be found in supplement form and in foods like yogurt and kefir. Recent studies suggest probiotics may be helpful in improving insulin sensitivity and reducing inflammation in people with diabetes. More research is needed, but in the meantime, try adding these foods to your meal plan.

8 Beyond the Flu Shot

August is Immunization Awareness Month. Aside from an annual flu shot, most adults with diabetes should also have the following vaccines: Tdap (tetanus, diphtheria, and whooping cough), pneumococcal (pneumonia), and hepatitis B. You may need additional immunizations based on your age, health, and the vaccines you had as a child.

9 The Problem with Pedicures

People with diabetes are prone to infection and foot problems, and this is why pedicures are not recommended. If you must get a pedicure, go to a reputable nail salon where equipment is sterilized and footbaths are disinfected before each use. Tell the nail tech to keep water temps cool, skip any callous filing, and leave cuticles alone. And never get a pedicure if you have any cuts or abrasions on your feet; the risk of further injury or infection is just too high.

10 Eat as a Family

Whenever possible, set the table and have the whole family sit down to dinner. Not only does it give you the opportunity to catch up with the people you love, but studies show that people who eat as a family eat more veggies and are less likely to be overweight—both important factors for people with diabetes.

11 Fruit on the Barbie

Save a spot on the grill for summer fruit favorites. A kabob of watermelon or peaches tastes great and is a refreshing twist on the usual barbecue fare. Grilling will caramelize the natural sugar in the fruit and bring out the flavor.

12 Beware of Leg Cramps

If you regularly get aching or cramping pain in your calves, buttocks, or thighs when walking or exercising, let your doctor know right away. It could be intermittent claudication caused by peripheral vascular disease (PVD). PVD is a narrowing of the arteries of the legs and feet. It can be controlled with medication, and regular exercise may actually help with the pain but should be supervised by a doctor.

13 Making the Shoe Fit

If you have any degree of neuropathy in your feet or other foot problems, you should see a licensed pedorthist for a proper shoe fitting. You may need prescription in-depth shoes. These shoes have an extra ¼- to ½-inch depth to accommodate special custom-fitted inserts called orthotics that relieve foot pressure and absorb shock. The right type of shoe can prevent limb loss, so don't delay, make an appointment today.

14 Restaurants on the Road

Eating smart while on vacation or a business trip can be a challenge. When you have to eat at restaurants, try to choose chains where you know healthy choices are available. Check online for menus and nutritional information or phone ahead to know your options. Once there, don't be shy about asking your server questions. Many restaurants are happy to make substitutions to meet your dietary needs.

15 Portion Buzz Words

Restaurants often serve entrées in portions big enough to feed a family. When eating out, avoid menu items that use the following words to describe the portion size: jumbo, extra large, supreme, triple, double, or grande. Instead, look for these words: small plate, appetizer, lunch portion, kid's size, petite, or junior.

16 Testing Tip: Strip Savings

Blood sugar testing strips can be expensive. When selecting a meter, find out how much its test strips cost so you can factor that into your decision. You might find a lower-cost generic or store brand that suits your budget better. You should also check with your health insurer to find out if they will only cover specific brands.

17 Sharps Safety in the Home

Don't leave used lancets or syringes lying around. Even if you don't have small children, it's too easy for other house-hold members or visitors to get an unintentional needle stick injury. You can purchase a sharps disposal container at any drug store. Or just use a hard plastic or metal container (e.g., empty detergent bottle, coffee can).

18 Fruits in Season: Blueberries

It's blueberry season, so enjoy these antioxidant-packed treats. Blueberry consumption has been tied to a reduced risk of developing type 2 diabetes. Blueberries have also lowered blood glucose levels and improved insulin sensitivity in animal studies. Skip the baked goods and have this sweet treat fresh; one cup of berries has 21 grams of carbohydrates and 3.6 grams of fiber.

19 Always Be Prepared

Everyone with diabetes should have an emergency kit in case of disaster. Your kit should have two weeks worth of diabetes supplies, extra batteries to power any devices, a first aid kit, drinking water, and nonperishable snacks (e.g., juice boxes, canned food). Rotate your supplies regularly so nothing expires.

20 Salad Bar Savvy

Salad bars can be calorie and carb black holes. Here's how to do them right. Skip the pastas, puddings, and deli salads. Instead, load up on all the raw veggies you'd like, along with a protein punch of chicken or turkey breast. Instead of croutons, noodles, or bacon bits, opt for a sprinkle of sunflower seeds or sliced almonds to add crunch. Finally, bypass the mystery salad dressings and top your creation with a light drizzle of oil and vinegar.

21 Is Generic Right for You?

Generic versions of brand name drugs can save you money. The Federal Drug Administration requires that generic drugs be just as safe and effective as brand name versions. Not all diabetes drugs have generic versions, but some do; ask your doctor or pharmacist if generic is an option for you.

22 When Family and Friends Don't Get It

It's hard when those around you either don't understand what you have to do to take care of your diabetes, or are completely misinformed about the disease. Consider bringing immediate family members or close friends along to a diabetes education class with you. Often, guests are allowed free of charge, and they can get a dose of real education as well as a better understanding of the challenges you face each day.

23 Portion Distortion

As consumers, we tend to underestimate calories and overestimate portion sizes. Studies show that what the average person thinks is a portion is usually about 20 percent larger than an actual serving. In addition, the larger the portions get, the more likely we are to underestimate the number of calories in a meal. Invest in a good kitchen scale to make sure your portions (and calories and carbs) are on target with reality.

24 Splitting "Peakless" Insulin

Long-acting insulin is designed to work for 24 hours without the "peak" in action other types of insulin provide. Although some long-acting insulin brands are designed for one dose daily, many people find that splitting their dose in two (morning and evening) provides better control. Ask your doctor if split dosing of your long-acting insulin might be right for you.

25 Fast and Slow Insulin Sites

Insulin injected into the abdomen works fastest, and insulin injected into the buttocks works the slowest. If you are taking a pre-meal injection, you may want to do it in the abdomen to quickly cover your carbohydrates. If you are taking insulin at night, you may want to choose the buttocks or thighs for a more gradual release.

26 Rotating Injections

If you are constantly injecting your insulin into the same spot on your body, it can cause your insulin to be less effective. If you can feel hard lumps or see "dents" at spots where you frequently inject, you may have lipodystrophy, or damage to the subcutaneous fat layer that affects how your insulin works. Always rotate sites at least an inch with each injection.

27 Fat and Your Blood Sugar

Foods that are high in fat and carbohydrates, such as ice cream or donuts, can cause a delayed blood glucose spike. The fat slows the absorption of carbohydrates, so your blood sugar may be near normal two to three hours after eating but suddenly skyrocket for up to 8 hours afterward.

28 Smart Bedtime Snacks

Eating a bedtime snack that includes some fat and protein can help keep your blood sugars even during the overnight hours. The fat and protein will both delay the carbohydrate absorption, and the protein will also help you feel satisfied. Reduced-fat string cheese, Greek yogurt, or whole grain crackers and natural peanut butter are all good choices. Snacks should be around 15 grams of carbohydrates each.

29 Skip the Rubbing Alcohol

There's no need to use rubbing alcohol to clean the skin before you do a finger stick or injection. It dries out your skin and there's no added benefit as long as your skin is clean. If you are testing, soap and water will do to clean your hands. If you do choose to use an alcohol swab, know that it will sting unless you make sure it's dry before puncturing the skin.

30 Medicinal Massage

Why not treat yourself to a massage today? In addition to feeling great, massage therapy can lower stress levels and blood pressure in people with hypertension. And studies show that it can improve blood circulation in people with type 2 diabetes and peripheral arterial disease (PAD).

31 Klutz-Proof Your Home

In an ideal world, people with diabetes would wear protective shoes both outside and inside the house. But in reality, at least in the summer months, you will probably barefoot it occasionally inside your home. If that's the case, make sure your home is safe to prevent foot injury. Clear stair and floor clutter daily. Secure all throw rugs or remove them completely, and light hallways with nightlights to prevent late night accidents.

September

It's a new school year for kids, and a great time to focus on your own diabetes education and habits. Pack a smarter lunch, try a new food, or pick up a new healthy hobby, such as yoga or brain training. Read on for more ideas.

1 Back to School

If it's been more than a year since you've visited a certified diabetes educator, sign up for an individual session or group class. Focus on a diabetes management skill you may be weak with, or just commit to learning one new thing. Remember, treatment and technology change quickly, and the only way to keep up is to educate yourself.

2 Brown Bag It

Packing lunch for work can save you time and money while improving your diabetes health. All it takes is a little planning and prep work. Pack up fresh favorites and vary your menu so lunch is something to look forward to. Try to avoid bringing in packaged frozen entrées—not only are they usually loaded with added sodium, but since they keep forever it can be tempting to skip out on the frozen food and hit a restaurant instead.

3 Better Bread Choices: Read the Label

The healthiest breads should always have a whole grain as the first ingredient listed on the label. Check the nutrition facts for those that are high in fiber and low in total carbohydrates. Remember, one serving is usually considered one slice, not two, so check the label.

4 Wrapping Up Lunch

Whole grain wraps or tortillas are a great, lower-carb substitute for bread. Again, choose those with a whole grain as one of the first ingredients. And here's a trick we love. Cut the bottom third off the wrap before placing your toppings and rolling it up. You'll still have plenty of wrap to hold your sandwich fixings in, but one third fewer carbs and calories.

5. Bread Cheats

If wraps aren't your thing, or you just can't part with your bread, never fear. An open-faced sandwich is a great carb-cutting strategy. So are thin sliced breads (just check the label for the nutritional values). Sourdough bread is also a smart choice, as it is known for having less of an impact on after-meal blood sugar levels than other breads.

6. Veggies in Season: Broccoli

This cruciferous veggie is filling and full of vitamin C, folate, potassium, and fiber. Try it steamed, in a stir-fry, grated up into a crunchy coleslaw, or as a raw snack.

7. Sandwiches on Ice

If you find yourself not packing lunch due to time constraints, here's a great idea. Spend a half hour each week prepping sandwiches. Store them in a freezer-safe wrap or container, and stow them until you need them. Just remember to avoid egg salad, which doesn't freeze well, and add any lettuce, tomato, and pickles after thawing.

8. You Aren't Your Neighbor's Diabetes

Blood sugar goals are not one-size-fits-all. Your goals may be very different than your next-door neighbor who is 85 years old and has COPD, or your pregnant daughter-in-law. Health history, age, other chronic health conditions, and other factors all play a part in what your goal should be. So get your A1C and testing goals from your health care team and try not to measure your "success" against other's individual goals.

9. Protect Your Bones

Type 1 diabetes raises the risk of developing osteoporosis, and type 2 diabetes is associated with an increased incidence of fractures. Protect your bones by getting plenty of dietary calcium in the form of green leafy veggies and dairy products.

If your doctor recommends calcium supplements, ask if you should be taking Vitamin D as well (which helps you absorb the calcium).

10 Veggie Up Your Breakfast

You may be having veggies at lunch and dinner and still not be getting your recommended 2 to 3 cups daily. Try adding veggies to your breakfast table, too. A little spinach in your eggs, a few slices of tomato on a breakfast wrap, or a glass of fresh homemade veggie juice all count toward your daily goal.

11 If the Shoe Fits

Never shop for shoes first thing in the morning. Your feet will swell throughout the day with activity, so a shoe that fits well early in the day may feel tight by late afternoon. Get both of your feet sized each time you shoe shop, and make sure shoes you try on are wide enough in the toe box to prevent crowding or pinching.

12 Downward Facing Diabetes

September is National Yoga Awareness Month. Did you know that studies have shown that the regular practice of yoga helps improve blood sugar control and lipid levels in people with diabetes? It's a great way to get active and reduce stress, especially if you are new to exercise. If you aren't aware of yoga classes in your area, ask at your community center or YMCA, or check out a yoga video online or at your local library.

13 Bring On the Bento Box

Replace your brown bag with a reusable bento box. These sectioned, preportioned containers are great for keeping portion sizes in check and encouraging you to include a variety of foods in your lunch. They also just look cool. Bento boxes are available in microwave-safe materials, so you can enjoy cold and hot foods together.

14 Lowering Your Stress Levels

Studies show that stress management programs can be highly effective in improving your mental outlook and your diabetes control. A Duke University study found that just five sessions of stress management training lowered A1C levels an average of half a percentage point. Meditation, music, art, and journaling are all proven stress-busting practices. Pick one you like and start doing it daily.

15 Why Whole Grains Matter

The whole grain is just that—the entire grain (bran, germ, and endosperm). Refined grains usually only contain the endosperm, which is the starchy and less nutritious part of the grain. It's the bran and germ that contain the protein, B vitamins, minerals, and fiber that are an important part of a healthy diet. Buckwheat, whole wheat, quinoa, millet, corn, wild rice, and rye are just a few tasty whole grain choices you can try adding to your menu today.

16 Testing Tip: Control Solution

Control solution is liquid that is used to calibrate your meter and make sure it's working properly and displaying correct test results. Not all meters require control solution, but if yours does, you need to know how it works and how often to use it. Read the directions for use for your meter to learn more.

17 Perfect Popcorn

Did you know popcorn is a whole grain? You can save money and make a healthier snack by popping your own corn. You'll also slash your sodium intake when you bypass the microwave popcorn. Add flavor by tossing popcorn with a small amount of Parmesan cheese or chili or garlic powder. Remember that portion control is important in keeping carbs in check, so serve in small bowls.

18 Fruits in Season: Guava

This often overlooked fruit can be consumed whole, including the rind and seeds. It's sweet, slightly acidic, and packed with potassium and antioxidants. One medium guava fruit is only 60 calories, 13 grams of carbohydrates, and 5 grams of fiber. If your local supermarket doesn't carry guava, try a Latin market.

19 How Lows Can Hurt Your Brain

Frequent episodes of hypoglycemia, or low blood sugar, have been associated with cognitive impairment in seniors with type 2. If you are experiencing memory or thinking problems and you are having a lot of lows, ask your doctor if a slightly higher A1C goal may be right for you.

20 Staying Sharp

It's normal to occasionally forget things, but as we age this can start to happen more frequently. Brain-stretching word games such as Sudoku, Scrabble, and crossword puzzles can keep your mental muscles strong. So pick up a puzzle book or app and make it a daily workout for your mind.

21 Beef on a Budget

Bonus money and time-saving fact—the toughest and least expensive cuts of meat become tender and tasty after hours of slow cooking. Buy chuck, brisket, round, flank, or skirt cuts of beef and pop them in a slow cooker with your favorite low-carb veggies for a delicious, no fuss dinner.

22 Fasting and Diabetes

Religious observances, such as Yom Kippur and Ramadan, involve fasting. If you take insulin, have problems with hypoglycemia, or have other health issues along with your diabetes, it may not be a good idea to fast. Ask your doctor, and then talk to your religious leader. Religions do have exemptions from fasting for those whose health might be put at risk by the practice.

23 Food Safety and Temperature

Whether you're bringing food home from the grocery store or taking a dish to a potluck, proper food transport temperatures are critical. Cold food needs to be kept at 40°F or lower. Hot foods should be at 140°F or higher. Temperatures outside of these ranges can breed bacteria and cause serious foodborne illnesses. Use insulated bags and heating or cooling packs to help keep the cold or heat in.

24 Get Up and Move

The American Diabetes Association recommends that people with diabetes break up any extended periods of inactivity (defined as 90 minutes or longer) with walking or other movement. So if you are sitting down to work, study, or do any other sedentary activity, set your phone or watch alarm to buzz you on the hour, then take a brisk walk.

25 Rethink Your Breakfast Drink

Drop the fruit juice and cut 100 to 200 calories from breakfast. Love the fruity flavor? Try squeezing a little fresh lemon or lime juice into your water instead, or add just a splash of orange or cranberry juice to sparkling water.

26 Fielding Fall Allergies

Fall is here, and if you have allergies, that also means ragweed, leaf fungus, and a whole lot of sneezing. Be careful with nasal sprays containing steroids, as these can raise blood sugar levels. And if you also have high blood pressure, avoid decongestants. Your best bet is to talk to your doctor or pharmacist for a recommendation on allergy medication that's safe for you.

27 Magic Noodles

Shirataki noodles are very low in calories and carbs, and high in a soluble fiber called glucomannan that comes from the root of the Japanese Konnyaku (or Konjac) plant. This high fiber content promotes feelings of fullness. Shirataki noodles come precooked in liquid and have a very chewy texture. There are also versions available that have tofu added for a smoother, less rubbery feel. Try them in Asian style stir-fries and soups.

28 Meter Readers

Ever find different blood sugar meters giving you very different test results? Food and Drug Administration regulations allow home blood glucose meters to be as much as 15% lower or higher than laboratory standards. If you ever feel high or low but your meter says your test results are in target, test again or try a different meter.

29 Carb-Conscious Cereal Choices

Love breakfast cereal but hate what it does to your blood sugar levels? Roll past the sugar-sweetened brands and opt for whole grain choices. Some good options include steel cut oatmeal, muesli, and unsweetened shredded wheat or bran cereal.

30 It's National Coffee Day!

Coffee lovers rejoice. That morning cup of java is good for your diabetes. Studies show coffee improves insulin sensitivity and glucose metabolism. As with most things, moderation is important. Limit yourself to two to three cups a day in the morning or early afternoon; evening coffee can keep you from a good night's sleep.

October

It's the scariest month of the year, but never fear ... we have tips to get you through the candy, cold weather, and other challenges of October.

1 Open Season

October means the start of open enrollment for health insurance for many Americans. Because your health and family are also changing, it's a good idea to reevaluate your options each year and make sure you have the best plan for managing your diabetes. If you get insurance through your employer, schedule an appointment with your benefits counselor to review your options.

2 FSAs and HSAs

Open enrollment month is also your chance to start planning for next year's health expenses. There are two options available: the flexible spending account (FSA) and the health savings account (HSA). These are a great way to save tax dollars on your diabetes expenses. Each offers different advantages, depending on your anticipated health spending needs in the coming year. Ask your accountant and/or your human resources representative about what may be right for you.

3 Schedule Your Flu Shot

Everyone with diabetes should get a flu shot early in the season. Diabetes puts you at higher risk for serious complications from the flu. To keep your home healthy, others in your household should also be sure to get flu shots. Schedule a flu shot today!

4 Souper Starts

It's soup season, so start your meal with a warm bowl of hearty soup. Soup is a great way to get more veggies into your diet. It also promotes satiety, or fullness, so when you start your meal with soup you are less likely to overeat.

5 The Leaf Pile Workout

If your weight is about 155 pounds, you can burn approximately 298 calories in just one hour by raking the lawn and sacking leaves. When you rake leaves, change your movement. Rake right to left and then left to right. You'll build up your arm muscles while you burn calories! This is a great way to add some variety to your workouts and get some vitamin D from the sun while you're outside.

6 Veggies in Season: Cabbage

Cabbage is a cruciferous veggie high in vitamins C and K and full of cancer-fighting, immunity-boosting antioxidants. A half cup of cabbage has only 4 grams of carbohydrates and 17 calories (along with 1 gram each of fiber and protein), making it a great choice for people with diabetes. Try it in an Oktoberfest sauerkraut, sliced up in slaw, or roasted and drizzled with olive oil.

7 Vitamin K and Blood Thinners

If you are on blood thinners, such as Coumadin (warfarin), you need to watch your vitamin K intake. That means not overdoing vitamin K rich foods, such as cabbage, spinach, broccoli, and many other leafy green veggies. The most important thing is to be consistent in your day-to-day intake of vitamin K.

8 Operation Identification

An ID bracelet, necklace, or other form of ID that says you have diabetes can be a lifesaver if you ever have a medical emergency. But it only works if you wear it. Never take it off when you exercise, as this is a high-risk time for a blood sugar emergency. There are so many comfortable and stylish options available for medical identification today that there's no good reason not to protect yourself.

9 Don't Buy Treats in Bulk

It's fine to have an occasional treat as part of your healthy meal plan. But your best bet is to buy small. Don't bring home economy size packages of cookies, chips, or other indulgences. But if you do end up with extra, freeze what's left over or store it away out of sight. Better yet, get it out of the house and share it with your coworkers or neighbors.

10 Vending Machines: Best Choices

Most of the time, a vending machine is not your best source of a nutritious snack. But there are times when it may be your only option. Opt for the peanuts or other nut options (e.g., trail mix). Sunflower seeds (kernel or whole) are also a great choice. Baked chips, pretzels, or popcorn will also do in a pinch, but will have more carbs. Skip the candy completely (unless needed to treat a low).

11 Label Lingo: Sell-By Dates

The "sell-by date" on a food label is the last date the store should keep the product on the shelf and available for sale. Remember that stores rotate their newer stock toward the back of shelves and coolers, so that's where you'll find the foods with the longest remaining shelf life. Once home, foods should be consumed within a few days of the sell-by date.

12 Fermented Foods as Spike Stoppers

Did you know that fermented and pickled foods, such as sauerkraut and kimchi, can help control post-meal blood sugar spikes? In addition, the acetic acid in these foods also helps contribute to a feeling of fullness. Try adding these to your lunch and dinner repertoire and see if your blood sugars respond. One note—when choosing pickles, skip the sweet varieties as these may have the opposite effect.

13 Medicine and Blood Sugar

Many nondiabetes medicines—both prescription and over-the-counter—can influence your blood sugar levels. When you get a new prescription, always ask your doctor how it might impact your diabetes. The pharmacist is a good source of information as well, especially if you are looking for over-the-counter medicines to treat a cold or other minor ailment.

14 Chronic Infections and Blood Sugar

Sugar makes an ideal breeding ground for bacteria. This is why people with uncontrolled or undiagnosed diabetes are more likely to develop infections of all types—from urinary tract and yeast infections to skin and oral infections. If you are getting lots of infections, it probably means your current diabetes treatment routine needs adjusting. Talk to your doctor about changes in medicine, and don't try to self-treat chronic infections.

15 A Smart Start to the Day

Your morning routine sets the tone for the entire day. Take 30 to 60 minutes the night before each work or school day to prep your lunch and snacks, pick your outfit, and take care of any other details you can do in advance. This will give you more time in the morning to do what you need for your diabetes—check your blood sugar, have a healthy breakfast, and exercise.

16 Testing Tip: Apps

It seems there's an app for everything these days. And blood sugar tracking is no exception. If you find pen and paper logging of your blood sugar testing results a burden, try one of the hundreds of available apps for smartphones, computers, and tablets. Some meters have their own associated apps available for free; check the instructions for use to find out more.

17 Hypoglycemia and Fats

Fat delays the absorption of sugar. That's why candy bars, doughnuts, and other fat-heavy sweets aren't a great choice for treating a low blood sugar episode (although they'll do in a pinch if they are all that's available). Glucose tablets or gels are the best choice because they work quickly. Keep a package in your pocket or handbag, the car, your desk, and anywhere else you can access them quickly if needed.

18 Fruits in Season: Apples

It's apple picking time. A small apple has 20.5 grams of carbo-hydrates, so when you indulge in this seasonal treat, plan the rest of your meal or snack accordingly. Apples also contain 3.6 grams of fiber and are high in vitamin C. To get all the nutritional benefits, eat the whole fruit versus applesauce and other derivatives.

19 Perfectly Packed Leftovers

The next time you make a casserole, stew, or other family entrée that results in leftovers, don't just put the whole pot or dish back into the fridge. Instead, pack the remainder in individ-ual size containers with a single portion in each. The fridge is fine for one or two containers that will be eaten within the next 24 to 48 hours, but freeze the rest to avoid any wasted food. When everything is preportioned, you are less likely to overeat.

20 How to Recalibrate Your Sleep Clock

Sleep deprivation can make your diabetes harder to control. If you work nights, here's how to get your body on a regu-lar sleep schedule. Wear dark sunglasses on your commute home and go to sleep immediately (don't be tempted by TV or chores). Use blackout curtains to keep your bedroom dark and cover up electronic sources of light, such as clocks. And make sure you get plenty of exposure to bright light during your waking and working hours to shift your circadian sleep cycle.

21 Wiping Out Bloodstains

Finger sticks and insulin injections mean you may occasion-ally get a blood drop on your clothing. Remember that a wet bloodstain is easier to remove than a dry one, so whenever possible immediately run cold water over the stain. A bit of salt or saline solution can help loosen it further. If the stain persists, or you discover a stain that has already dried, a weak hydrogen peroxide solution will usually do the trick.

22 Spaghetti Squash Swap

Spaghetti squash topped with marinara makes a delicious lower-carb alternative to traditional spaghetti. Just bake or roast the squash, scrape out the spaghetti-like squash strands, and toss with marinara. When you choose a sauce, check the label for a version without added sugar.

23 Pasta Perfection

If you are a die-hard pasta lover, try whole grain versions that are high in insoluble fiber and may have less of an impact on your blood sugar levels. Remember, al dente pasta (pasta cooked "firm to the tooth") has a lower glycemic index than well-cooked pasta.

24 Hidden Carbs in Soups and Stews

Thickeners, such as flour and cornstarch, can add a lot of carbohydrates to your soups and stews. When ordering at restaurants, don't hesitate to ask your waitress if thickeners were used in the soup. If you are making homemade soup, try pureed veggies, sour cream, or almond meal for thickening without all the added carbs.

25 More Smart Soups

And speaking of soups ... what are the best options? Again, veggies rule the day for nutrient value and carbohydrate kindness. Broth-based soups, such as vegetable and minestrone (minus the pasta), are a good choice. So are those starring pureed veggies, such as tomato and squash.

26 Getting Past Diabetes Fears

Diabetes can be scary. You may be afraid of getting complications or of dying early. Here's the thing you need to remember. Diabetic complications are *not* inevitable. If you do the right things to manage your blood sugar levels, they are likely to be preventable and in some cases reversible. And the healthy lifestyle you must lead to control your diabetes means that you are probably on target to live a longer, healthier life than many of your peers without diabetes.

27 Shop the Perimeter

You can find the healthiest foods around the perimeter of your grocery store. That's where you'll find vegetables, fruits, lean proteins (chicken and fish), and dairy products. You can skip the bakery corner of the store, unless you're stopping for whole grain bread. And visit the inner aisles only to retrieve items you have put on a shopping list beforehand.

28 Keeping Things in Perspective

Diabetes can be hard, and sometimes all the testing, carb counting, and medication management feels overwhelming. If it feels like you are taking on too much, pick one thing to focus on for now. Schedule an appointment with your certified diabetes educator, who can help you to prioritize your diabetes management. And get involved with a diabetes support group so you can have a place to vent with people who "get it."

29 The Power of Pumpkin

Pumpkins are everywhere this time of year, so it's a great time to work this superfood into your daily diet. Pumpkins are high in fiber and packed with healthy beta carotene, which is good for your vision and helps protect your immune system. There is also some animal research that indicates they may contain substances that help control blood sugar. In addition to pumpkin breads and desserts, which can be carb heavy, pumpkin tastes great in soups and stews.

30 Perfect Pepitas

October is also a great month for roasted pumpkin seeds, or pepitas. These crunchy treats are chock full of protein, copper, magnesium, zinc, and more. Just remember to watch portions—they are high in fat, so the calories can add up.

31 Avoiding Halloween Horrors

If you hand out treats for Halloween, you know the siren song of the Fun Sized candy bar. Eat a healthy and filling meal before trick-or-treaters start descending to avoid the temptation of the candy bowl. And if you have leftovers, get them all out of the house the following morning. Donate to operationshoebox.com or halloweencandybuyback.com and your treats will make their way to a soldier overseas.

November

Diabetes is in the spotlight this month as Americans observe National Diabetes Month. Mark the occasion by learning more about advocacy and spreading a little diabetes awareness. We also have tips to help you through seasonal stresses with the kickoff of the holidays at Thanksgiving.

1. Wearing Blue for Diabetes

Blue is the official color of diabetes awareness. The group Diabetes Social Media Advocacy started the "Blue Friday" movement to bring attention to World Diabetes Day (November 14) and the disease of diabetes. So every Friday, wear your blue with pride. Be creative! Wear a blue hat and gloves over the winter and blue sunglasses or sneakers during the warmer months.

2. Team Up to Tame Holiday Stress

A daily walk with a friend or coworker is a great way to reduce stress, lift your mood, and stay healthy at the same time. You can chat while you walk for even more emotional support if you are feeling overwhelmed. It's a great way to support each other without focusing on food or other commitments during this very busy and potentially stressful time of year.

3. Recognizing Depression

If you have diabetes, you are at higher risk for depression. Keep your eye out for signs of depression, such as changes in appetite or sleep patterns, loss of energy, lack of interest in things that you used to enjoy, hopeless feelings, and an inability to complete daily tasks. If you are feeling depressed, tell your doctor. Medication and/or therapy can help. So can learning more about taking care of your diabetes properly through a diabetes self-management education program.

4. Recognizing Depression in Older Adults

As we get older, we may not necessarily feel sad when we are depressed, but we may feel helpless. Other signs, such as an intense lack of motivation, unexplained aches and pains, and a decline in grooming behaviors (e.g., not showering) are common. Your health care provider can offer support and treatment so you can live a happier and healthier life. Review your current medications with your doctor as well, because some may worsen symptoms of depression.

5 Veggies in Season: Red Cabbage

Colorful red cabbage is a delicious addition to any salad, vegetable dish, or soup. Try stir-frying red cabbage in a little olive oil and topping it with cinnamon, nutmeg, walnuts, and a chopped apple for a luscious treat. One full cup of chopped red cabbage has only 28 calories and 7 grams of carbohydrates, and it is a good source of antioxidants, fiber, and vitamins C, A, and K.

6 Navigating Buffets

Before you join the buffet line, walk around once to see the offerings. This will prevent you from filling your plate with the first items you see and overeating on dishes that you don't really enjoy. Make sure to focus on colorful vegetables and lean protein, such as fish, chicken, or turkey. If you decide to eat a particular dish (or dessert) that is high in carbs or calories, eat only one serving and enjoy it!

7 Buffets, Take Two

One of the biggest problems with most buffets is that they allow you to return and refill your plate as many times as you like. Limit yourself to one trip for a healthy green salad and one for your main meal. Using the smaller, salad size plates for both visits can help you manage your portion sizes. Have a large glass of water along with each plate and you should be full enough to sidestep the bottomless buffet pitfall.

8 Notes on Noshing

If you've ever walked through a grocery store on "sample day," you know it's a minefield of different processed food items. Even if you manage to bypass samples, the deli clerk will hand you slices of cheese and meat while you're waiting for your order to be ready. All of these little nibbles and noshes can add up to a lot of extra calories and carbs (not to mention salt and extra fat). Calories count even if you're pushing a shopping cart, so make sure you are mindful of what you put in your mouth.

9 | Mind Your Own Plate

Never eat off of anyone else's plate. If your child or dining companion doesn't finish their meal, then pack it up as leftovers or toss it into the garbage. It's better off there than in your body as additional calories and carbohydrates.

10 | Gearing Up for Cold Weather Exercise

Dress for winter exercise success! Wear a thin layer of synthetic material next to your body, such as polypropylene. This material draws moisture (or sweat) away from your body, so it's perfect for outdoor workouts. You can wear additional layers over that, and remove them for comfort while exercising. Wear a hat, earmuffs, and gloves to protect your head, ears, and hands from the elements.

11 | Winter Outdoor Exercise Safety

Keep your supplies and/or insulin under your clothing or in a portable pack that will prevent these lifesaving items from freezing. Always drink plenty of water to stay hydrated, even if you don't feel thirsty. Be aware of the signs and symptoms of hypothermia and hypoglycemia, and always check your blood sugar before, during, and after your workouts.

12 | Warm Drinks for Cold Days

There is nothing like a warm cup of soothing tea on a cold winter day. Green tea is high in antioxidants and tastes great, even without added sweetener. Opt for the decaf versions if it's later in the day. Or try flavored herb or spiced decaffeinated teas for a tasty treat anytime of the day or evening. If you want something savory, enjoy a cup of reduced-sodium broth. This hot beverage is low in calories and is very satisfying.

13 | Beating Diabetes Burnout

Your diabetes never takes a day off, even when you need a break from taking care of it. If you notice yourself starting to miss blood sugar tests, medications, and other important diabetes tasks, you may be experiencing diabetes burnout. Take a moment to reach out to others for support. It's also important to speak to your doctor or certified diabetes educator about ways to make your diabetes more manageable for you and your lifestyle.

14 It's World Diabetes Day

Led by the International Diabetes Foundation, World Diabetes Day was started in 1991 to create a global voice of diabetes advocacy and awareness. You are your own best advocate for improving life with diabetes. Observe the day by getting involved with a local diabetes advocacy group to share your experiences and gain support from others. Both the American Diabetes Association (ADA) and JDRF have local chapters across America.

15 Invest In a Cure

The Diabetes Research Institute, the Joslin Diabetes Center, and the UC San Diego Diabetes Research Center are just a few of many organizations working on cutting-edge research toward finding a cure for diabetes. Learn more about their missions and support one or more of these organizations through the many volunteer or fund-raising opportunities their foundations offer.

16 Social Media Support

The diabetes online community (DOC) is a way for people with diabetes around the world to form communities, share information with others, and discuss experiences. Conversations are shared through blogs, Twitter, Facebook, and other online forums. Once you become more comfortable with social media, you may feel ready to join the discussion.

17 It's National "Take a Hike" Day

Changing your "exercise scenery" can be truly motivating and exhilarating. Many towns have nature preserves with hiking access, or you can design your own walking path through nearby neighborhoods. Trail walking can be particularly good exercise if the terrain is varied. Become familiar with your path and plan the distance of your journey so that it will be safe and enjoyable.

18 Testing Tip: Always Have Clean Hands

Cleaning your fingers correctly before blood sugar testing is essential. Wash your hands with warm and soapy water and make sure to dry them before testing. If you eat something and then test your blood sugar without washing your hands, you may have an inaccurate blood sugar reading. Food residue may cause a high reading.

19 Stuffing Substitutes

Try almond flour instead of bread crumbs for your stuffing recipes. It will help soak up the liquids and add texture to the finished dish. Use lean chicken sausage instead of traditional sausage to cut back on extra fat calories. If your recipe calls for fruit juice, substitute fresh-squeezed lemon juice (cut with water) instead. Make sure to use low-sodium broth and plenty of seasoning and spices for added flavor, and toss in some walnuts for a boost of omega-3's.

20 Healthy Dessert Swaps

If you enjoy holiday baking, here are a few ways to lower carbohydrates in your baked goods. Try using cooked black beans (rinsed, drained, and pureed) for flour. Use 1 cup of black beans as a substitute for 1 cup of flour. You can also try whole wheat flour instead of white flour, but use a little less ($7/8$ cup to 1 cup of white flour). Nut flours are also an option, but look for recipes already tested with almond or other nut flours—substitutions can be tricky.

21 Talking Turkey

No need to slather your turkey in butter, just make sure you don't overcook it. If you cook it for the correct amount of time, and baste it repeatedly, it should come out moist and delicious. Use a low-sodium broth to supplement the natural juices for basting, and make sure to season it with plenty of onions, carrots, and mushrooms. A 3-ounce serving of turkey breast is only about 88 calories with 3.5 grams of carbohydrates.

22 Plant-Based Diets

Yes, you can follow a vegetarian or vegan eating plan safely and successfully with diabetes. Studies have shown that if planned correctly, a vegetarian diet can help promote weight loss and improve A1C levels for people with diabetes. If you are new to either diabetes or vegetarianism/veganism, it's important to see a registered dietitian nutritionist to learn how to balance carb intake and get enough protein.

23 The Smart Vegetarian

Even though they are healthy, don't forget that eating too many whole grains and fruits can put you over your carbohydrate budget. So watch your portions and continue to choose low-carb vegetarian and vegan options. Meat and poultry substitutes, such as veggie burgers, tempeh, or seitan, do provide vegetable-based protein, but also contain some carbohydrate and sodium. Always check nutrition labels and plan your meals accordingly.

24 Mocktails for the Holidays

Toast the holidays with different flavored seltzers poured into a wine glass or champagne flute for a toast. You'll still be social and save the extra calories and carbs (and prevent a low blood sugar) at the same time. Freeze cranberries and mint into ice cubes for a festive and fun garnish.

25 Protecting Thanksgiving Leftovers

Store leftovers in shallow, air tight containers to make sure food cools quickly and stays at 40°F or cooler when refrigerated or frozen. This will prevent bacterial growth. Make sure the lids fit securely on the containers so the food stays moist. When reheating, always use a meat thermometer to make sure foods are heated to a safe internal temperature (at least 165°F).

26 Stop Stress Eating

Did you know that chronic stress actually increases your appetite and makes you crave high-sugar, high-fat "comfort foods," which in turn promote weight gain? There is a reason they are called comfort foods, but while they may make you temporarily feel better, there is a long-term cost to your diabetes. A better stress-coping strategy? A quick workout. The endorphins released through exercise fight the negative effects of stress (and the workout is great for your diabetes, too).

27 Make Time for Yourself

It's important to make time for yourself each and every day to stay balanced and happy and cope with life's stresses. Put downtime into your daily schedule. Make this time a routine part of your day, and don't compromise. Do what you want to do during that 15 to 30 minutes. You can listen to your favorite tunes, read a newspaper, or call a friend.

28 Fruits in Season: Bananas

Bananas are a sweet, portable fruit, and come wrapped in their own neat package. They are a great source of potassium, which may be of benefit to people with high blood pressure. One medium banana has about 110 calories and 30 grams of carbohydrates, and half of a banana makes a sweet and satisfying snack. If you are planning on exercising for an extended period of time, have a banana first for an extra boost of carbohydrate energy.

29 De-stressing the Holidays: Making Your List

Keep your sanity this holiday season. Write a list of everything you want to get done (no task is too small). Remember to include the things that you *want* to do, not just what you *have* to do. And make sure it's realistic; you are allowed to eliminate any items that are adding stress without giving joy in return. This will help you stay organized and feel accomplished as you check items off on your list.

30 De-stressing the Holidays: Checking it Twice

Don't let taking care of yourself fall off your "to do" list this holiday. Keep up with your exercise schedule to keep stress and weight under control. One way to ensure you take time out to battle holiday stress is to pick up the phone now and book a massage or other spa treat in the weeks leading up to holiday gatherings. Pay up front so you won't cancel at the last minute.

December

The last month of the year can be the most challenging for many people with diabetes. It's a time of joy, but it can also be a time of great stress as you travel, shop, drink, and eat your way through the season. The good news is there are simple, small changes you can make to bring a healthier spin to your holiday favorites.

1 Pie Day

December 1st is National Pie Day (yes, there's a day for everything). Here are a few ideas to make your favorite holiday pies healthier. First, cut the carbohydrates by using only a bottom or a top crust, not both. Or experiment with whole wheat or nut flours in making your crust. Instead of sugar, try no-calorie sweetener mixes made for baking, and use sweeter spices such as cinnamon, nutmeg, ginger, and vanilla to add flavor without carbs.

2 Holiday Hosting Tips

Hosting a holiday gathering? Most of the time the host is so busy with tending to guests that overindulging isn't a problem. But preparing for a party can lead you into food temptations, especially if you are cooking up a variety of holiday favorites. Eat a healthy meal before you start cooking so you won't find yourself mindlessly munching through the day. Or consider catering the event, and send each guest home with a "doggie bag" tray of the leftovers.

3 Being the Perfect Guest

Holiday parties are great fun, but they can also be a challenge if you are trying to manage your blood sugar. It helps to eat a healthy meal before you go to an event that's centered around drinks and desserts, then pick one indulgence to treat yourself to. If it's a dinner party, your contribution can be a lower-carb dish you know you can eat. Just let the hosts know ahead of time—most will appreciate the gesture (and other guests probably will, too).

4 Baking with Sugar Substitutes

Sugar does more than sweeten baked goods; it also helps them with rising, browning, and texture. That's why replacing sugar directly with a non-caloric table sweetener isn't always successful. Instead, try blends formulated for baking, which mix sweeteners with a small amount of regular sugar to help with these important properties.

5 Low-Carb Coffee Drinks

Love your lattes? You can have your favorite flavored coffee drink without the added sugar. Many coffee chains usually carry at least one variety of sugar-free coffee syrups. Just ask what your options are. Or you can purchase your own sugar-free syrups for use at home. DaVinci and Torani are two brands that offer a full line of sugar-free flavors, including chocolate, gingerbread, and marshmallow.

6 Veggies in Season: Swiss Chard

Swiss chard is low in calories and carbohydrates and high in vitamins A, C, and K. Have it raw as a salad green, sauté it with a little olive oil, add it to soup, or mix it in a frittata or quiche. It's as versatile as it is delicious.

7 Restaurants by the Numbers

As of December 2015, federal law requires restaurants to label all menu items with calorie counts. The law applies to restaurants and any retail chain that serves ready-to-eat food and has 20 or more locations (e.g., movie theaters, convenience stores). Chains are also required to provide additional nutritional information (including carbohydrates) to any customer upon request. This is great news for all Americans trying to make healthier choices when they eat out.

8 Low-Carb Cookies

Meringue cookies are sinfully sweet and low in calories. They are also simple to make with few ingredients—egg whites, cream of tartar, and sugar. Just substitute the refined sugar with a sweetener blend such as Splenda Sugar Blend for Baking to lower the carbohydrate count. If you like to experiment with flavor, try a dash of almond, vanilla, coconut, or peppermint extract. You can also add a drop of food coloring to the mix for a cheerful holiday look.

9 Operation Medication Organization

If you are managing more than one chronic health condition, you may be taking many pills prescribed by several doctors. Each time you go to visit your diabetes doctor or certified diabetes educator (CDE), bring all of your prescription medicines, over-the-counter drugs, and supplements. Include the original packaging and labels. Your health care provider can review what you're taking and make sure none of your medicines are causing problems with your blood sugar control.

10 Tea Time

Did you know that brewed green tea may actually help your diabetes health? Some research shows that green tea can improve insulin resistance, reduce fasting glucose levels, and reduce A1C. Remember that green tea does have caffeine (although less than black tea or coffee), so be careful about consuming it too close to bedtime.

11 Make the Pharmacist Your Friend

It's a good idea to get all your prescriptions filled at one pharmacy. Choose a store or chain that tracks all of your medicines in a computer database and flags any potential drug interactions. And when you're shopping for supplements or over-the-counter remedies, enlist the pharmacist for help. He can help guide you toward choices that won't interact with your other medicines and are safe for your diabetes.

12 Own Your Health Care

When you go for diabetes-related lab work, always request that a copy of the results be sent to you. If your provider or lab service has an electronic health records portal for patients, this can be a fast and easy way to access results. If you don't understand what certain lab results mean, call the doctor or bring the report to your next appointment and ask.

13 The Fat Free Follies

Be wary of snack foods that are labeled "fat free." Behavioral research has shown that people tend to overeat these foods; they perceive these foods as guilt-free indulgences, and they also think serving sizes of these foods are larger than they really are. In addition, many fat-free foods can be higher in carbohydrates than their full-fat equivalents. Bottom line: always read the nutrition label before you buy.

14 Toasty Tootsies

If you have diabetic neuropathy and/or circulation problems, your feet may be chronically cold, especially during the winter months. Never use hot water bottles or heating pads to keep feet warm in bed; you could burn yourself without knowing it. Instead, treat your feet to a pair of fuzzy and warm seamless socks.

15 Insulin and Exercise

If you take insulin, remember to never exercise right after an injection. Your body needs at least 90 minutes to metabolize the insulin. You should also avoid exercise during the time your insulin is peaking (when this is will depend on the type of insulin you take; ask your doctor if you aren't sure).

16 Testing Tip: Know Your Influencers

Your hematocrit level (the number of red blood cells you have) can affect your blood sugar testing results if it is too high or too low. Substances such as ascorbic acid (vitamin C), uric acid, and acetaminophen (Tylenol) can also affect readings. Talk to your doctor or CDE about how your health conditions or medicines could influence your blood sugar test results.

17 Seasonal Spritzers

Cut back on your alcohol consumption while still being festive by drinking a red or white wine spritzer this holiday season. If mixing for a party, mix one bottle (750 mL) dry red or white wine to one quart of sparkling water or seltzer. If you are mixing by the glass, go for half-and-half in a 5-ounce wine glass.

18 Fruits in Season: Cranberries

One study found that cranberries can reduce LDL and total cholesterol levels in people with type 2 diabetes. But skip sugar-laden cranberry sauces and jelly that will spike your blood sugar. Instead, opt for whole cranberries that add a tart twist to both sweet and savory dishes. Try a handful of cranberries cooked in to steel cut oatmeal, or roast cranberries with thyme and add them to whole grain wild rice.

19 Frozen Shoulder

Adhesive capsulitis, or frozen shoulder, is a diabetes complication that causes stiffening of the shoulder and can limit arm movement. Controlling your blood sugar is the best way to prevent frozen shoulder, since the condition is caused by glucose binding with the collagen in your shoulder. If you do develop frozen shoulder, getting a prompt diagnosis and treatment is important. Physical therapy can help return movement to normal, along with medications for pain and inflammation.

20 Family Faux Pas

Holiday time means gatherings with family you may not see very often, and who may not know a lot about diabetes care. And when you're sitting down to a table filled with holiday food, they may take it upon themselves to comment on everything you choose to eat. Take a deep breath and try to use the moment as a teaching opportunity. And remind yourself that you probably won't have to see them again until next December.

21 Cha-Cha-Cha-Chia Seeds

Chia seeds are more than just a "as seen on TV" novelty gift. These nutty-tasting super seeds are high in omega-3 fatty acids, calcium, iron, and fiber. Some research indicates that chia may be helpful in promoting feelings of satiety (fullness) and in moderating after-meal blood sugar levels. One tablespoon of chia seeds contains 60 calories, 5 grams of carbohydrates, and 5 grams of fiber. Sprinkle them on steamed veggies, swirl them into yogurt, or toss a spoonful into salad.

22 Flying and Diabetes

Always carry your blood sugar testing supplies and medication in your carry-on bag in case of lost luggage. When you go through security, let TSA personnel know what's in your bag. If you take insulin pens or syringes, bring the original prescription packaging for your insulin. Some people prefer to travel with a letter from their doctor stating that they have diabetes and they require insulin injections.

23 Flying with Medical Devices

If you wear an insulin pump and/or a continuous glucose monitor, tell the TSA agent. You should not have to disconnect to get through security, but the electromagnetic scanner in use at most TSA checkpoints can damage your medical equipment. Request a manual check, and if you run into problems, ask for a TSA supervisor.

24 Cuckoo for Cocoa

Love hot cocoa but don't like what it does to your blood sugar? A few smart swaps can help. Start with unsweetened cocoa powder and use unsweetened almond milk instead of milk or cream. Sweeten your cocoa to taste with your favorite no-calorie sweetener, or try a shot of sugar-free peppermint or marshmallow syrup.

25 Gifts of the Season

Give yourself the gift of time and enjoyment this season by dialing back on some of the holiday hoopla. Pick one or two holiday celebrations you'd like to attend instead of feeling obligated to accept every invitation. Ask your family for help with the decorating, cooking, and shopping. By saving yourself some of the extra stress that comes this time of year, you'll have a healthier, happier holiday.

26 Eating Out and Insulin

If you take before-meal insulin injections, be careful about injecting too early when eating out at restaurants. To avoid an unnecessary blood sugar low, always wait until the food is set down in front of you before you take your insulin. You never know when a busy night, a slow waitstaff, or a kitchen mix-up will delay your meal.

27 Check Your Shoes

It may sound a bit strange, but you should make it a habit to inspect the inside of your shoes or boots before you put them on every day. Give them a good shake to make sure there is nothing inside. If you have peripheral neuropathy in your feet, you may not feel an object in your shoes, and even a small pebble could cause a serious wound if you walk on it all day.

28 Managing Metformin Side Effects

Metformin can cause gastrointestinal side effects (e.g., nausea, diarrhea, and cramping) in some people. The medication is usually started at a low dose and then gradually increased over time to minimize side effects, which often decrease over time. If you are having unpleasant side effects from metformin that aren't improving, call your health care provider and ask if a dose adjustment can help.

29 A Word of Warning

Never stop taking a diabetes drug (or any other prescribed medicine) without first speaking with your health care provider. If the medicine is too expensive, or if side effects are a lingering problem, call your doctor and ask if there are other medication options for you. You and your health care team should work together to find a treatment that not only addresses the medical need but also fits your lifestyle.

30 Medicine is Not a Sign of Failure

Type 2 diabetes is a progressive disease. Insulin resistance increases with age, as does pancreatic beta cell death. Even with the most diligent attention to diet and other diabetes care, most people with type 2 will eventually require insulin, oral medicine, or other injectable diabetes medicines. This isn't a sign of failure, so never feel bad about "not beating your diabetes."

31 Ringing In the New Year

On New Year's Eve it's tempting to overdo the alcohol. Make sure you know what a drink actually is. One drink is a 5-ounce glass of wine, one 12-ounce beer, or a single shot (1.5 ounces) of distilled spirits. And keep in mind that men should limit themselves to two drinks a day, and women to one (thanks to differences in body composition). So save your quota for that midnight toast and start next year healthier and hangover-free.

Acknowledgments

We'd like to express our heartfelt appreciation to the incomparable Jim Turner for contributing his wit and wisdom to the Foreword of this book. We love you Jim. We are also grateful for the friendship and support of everyone in the diabetes community; you rise to the challenge of this disease every single day and have taught us both so much. Thanks to Julia Pastore for bringing this project to us and shepherding it through to publication, and to Michael O'Connor for the eagle eye he brought to the manuscript. And for keeping us entertained for decades and being an equal-opportunity diabetes employer, we say thanks and "Hey Now" to Howard Stern. Last but not least, Susan would like to thank her family and friends for their inspiration and endless love. And Paula would like to thank her family, near and far, for their love and support.

Notes

Chapter 1

p. 3 *Studies show that a loss* ... Jensen MD, Ryan DH, Apovian CM, et al. 2013 AHA/ACC/TOS guideline for the management of overweight and obesity in adults: a report of the American College of Cardiology/American Heart Association Task Force on Practice Guidelines and The Obesity Society. *J Am Coll Cardiol.* 2014;63(25_PA):2985–3023.

p. 7 *In addition to being full of fiber* ... Kirpitch AR, Melinda DM. The 3 R's of glycemic index: recommendations, research, and the real world. *Clin Diabetes.* 2011;29(4):155–159.

p. 8 *Recent research has found a connection* ... Izuora K, Ezeanolue E, Schlauch K, Neubauer M, Gewelber C, Umpierrez G. Impact of periodontal disease on outcomes in diabetes. *Contemp Clin Trials.* 2015;41C:93–99.

Chapter 2

p. 15 *The cocoa bean* ... Esser D, Mars M, Oosterink E, Stalmach A, Muller M, Afman LA. Dark chocolate consumption improves leukocyte adhesion factors and vascular function in overweight men. *FASEB J.* 2013;28(3):1464.

p. 17 *Prickly pears are the fruit* ... Cefalu WT, Stephens JM, Ribnicky DM. Diabetes and herbal (botanical) medicine. In: Benzie IFF, Wachtel-Galor S, eds. *Herbal Medicine: Biomolecular and Clinical Aspects.* 2nd ed. Boca Raton, FL: CRC Press; 2011; chap 19. Available at: www.ncbi.nlm.nih.gov/books/NBK92755. Accessed February 6, 2015.

p. 17 *Omega-3s are important* ... Abeywardena MY, Patten GS. Role of ω3 long-chain polyunsaturated fatty acids in reducing cardio-metabolic risk factors. *Endocr Metab Immune Disord Drug Targets.* 2011;11(3):232–246. Review.

p. 18 *Did you know that federal law* ... Americans With Disabilities Act of 1990. 42 U.S.C. §§ 12101 et seq.

Chapter 3

p. 23 *Studies show that people who eat while distracted* ... Wansink B. Environmental factors that increase the food intake and consumption volume of unknowing consumers. *Annu Rev Nutr.* 2004;24:455–479. Review.

p. 24 *At least once a year* ... American Diabetes Association. Standards of medical care in diabetes—2015. *Diabetes Care.* 2015;38(suppl. 1): S58-S66.

p. 24 *Studies show that the DASH program* ... Craddick SR, Elmer PJ, Obarzanek E, Vollmer WM, Svetkey LP, Swain MC. The DASH diet and blood pressure. *Curr Atheroscler Rep.* 2003;5(6):484–491.

p. 27 *Proper sleep is critical* ... Sheikh-Ali M, Maharaj J. Circadian clock desynchronisation and metabolic syndrome. *Postgrad Med J.* 2014;90(1066):461–466. doi: 10.1136/postgradmedj-2013–132366. Epub 2014 Jun 23.

p. 27 *Studies show that high daily water intake* ... Sontrop JM, Dixon SN, Garg AX. Association between water intake, chronic kidney disease, and cardiovascular disease: a cross-sectional analysis of NHANES data. *Am J Nephrol.* 2013;37(5):434–442.

p. 28 *The good news is that treating OSA* ... Grimaldi D, Beccuti G, Touma C, Van Cauter E, Mokhlesi B. Association of obstructive sleep apnea in rapid eye movement sleep with reduced glycemic control in type 2 diabetes: therapeutic implications. *Diabetes Care.* 2014;37(2):355–363.

p. 28 *Research shows that people often overeat* ... Robinson E, Aveyard P, Daley A, et al. Eating attentively: a systematic review and meta-analysis of the effect of food intake memory and awareness on eating. *Am J Clin Nutr.* 2013;97(4):728–742.

p. 30 *People with type 2 diabetes are at a higher risk* ... Berster JM, Göke B. Type 2 diabetes mellitus as risk factor for colorectal cancer. *Arch Physiol Biochem.* 2008;114(1):84–98.

Chapter 4

p. 34 *Canned tomatoes actually contain* ... USDA Agricultural Research Service. About Tomatoes and Lycopene. Available at: http://www.ars.usda.gov/Research/docs.htm?docid=19428. Accessed January 18, 2015.

p. 35 *Use small, shallow bowls* ... Wansink B, van Ittersum K. Portion size me: plate-size induced consumption norms and win-win solutions for reducing food intake and waste. *J Exp Psychol Appl.* 2013;19(4):320–332.

p. 36 *Try this type of exercise* ... Colberg SR, Sigal RJ, Fernhall B, et al. Exercise and type 2 diabetes: the American College of Sports Medicine and the American Diabetes Association: joint position statement. *Diabetes Care.* 2010;33(12):e147-e167. doi: 10.2337/dc10–9990.

p. 36 *Mushrooms are low in calories* ... Anderson GH, Soeandy CD, Smith CE. White vegetables: glycemia and satiety. *Adv Nutr.* 2013;4(3):356S-367S.

p. 36 *Mushrooms are low in calories* ... Jayasuriya WJ, Wanigatunge CA, Fernando GH, Abeytunga DT, Suresh TS. Hypoglycaemic activity of culinary *Pleurotus ostreatus* and *P. cystidiosus* mushrooms in healthy volunteers and type 2 diabetic patients on diet control and the possible mechanisms of action. *Phytother Res.* 2014.

p. 37 *Bromelain has anti-inflammatory* ... Bromelain. Monograph. *Altern Med Rev.* 2010;15(4):361–368. Review.

p. 37 *And that's good news for you* ... Padiya R, Banerjee SK. Garlic as an anti-diabetic agent: recent progress and patent reviews. *Recent Pat Food Nutr Agric.* 2013;5(2):105–127. Review.

p. 37 *And that's good news for you* ... Senthilkumar KS, Senthilkumar GP, Sankar P, Bobby Z. Attenuation of oxidative stress, inflammation and insulin resistance by allium sativum in fructose-fed male rats. *J Clin Diagn Res.* 2013;7(9):1860–1862.

p. 37 *Keeping the sleep environment* ... Fonken LK, Nelson RJ. The effects of light at night on circadian clocks and metabolism. *Endocr Rev.* 2014;35(4):648–670. doi: 10.1210/er.2013–1051.

p. 38 *When we don't sleep enough* ... Copinschi G, Leproult R, Spiegel K. The important role of sleep in metabolism. *Front Horm Res.* 2014;42:59–72.

Chapter 5

p. 43 *There is good research that shows* ... Ros E, Martínez-González MA, Estruch R, et al. Mediterranean diet and cardiovascular health: teachings of the PREDIMED study. *Adv Nutr.* 2014;5(3):330S-336S.

p. 43 *There is good research that shows* ... Grosso G, Buscemi S, Galvano F, et al. Mediterranean diet and cancer: epidemiological evidence and mechanism of selected aspects. *BMC Surg*. 2013;13 (suppl. 2):S14.

p. 43 *There is good research that shows* ... Koloverou E, Esposito K, Giugliano D, Panagiotakos D. The effect of Mediterranean diet on the development of type 2 diabetes mellitus: a meta-analysis of 10 prospective studies and 136,846 participants. *Metabolism*. 2014;63(7):903–911.

p. 44 *But research now tells us* ... Maclean PS, Bergouignan A, Cornier MA, Jackman MR. Biology's response to dieting: the impetus for weight regain. *Am J Physiol Regul Integr Comp Physiol*. 2011;301(3):R581-R600.

p. 44 *Anxiety is a common issue* ... Ducat L, Philipson LH, Anderson BJ. The mental health comorbidities of diabetes. *JAMA*. 2014;312(7):691–692.

p. 48 *Whole grains are a great source* ... Wu H, Flint AJ, Qi Q, et al. Association between dietary whole grain intake and risk of mortality: two large prospective studies in US men and women. *JAMA Intern Med*. 2015;175(3):373–384.

p. 48 *If you have already gone gluten free* ... Kelly CP. Diagnosis of Celiac Disease. UpToDate. Oct 15, 2014. http://www.uptodate.com/contents/diagnosis-of-celiac-disease. Accessed February 8, 2015.

Chapter 6

p. 53 *Discuss your options* ... Grossmann M. Testosterone and glucose metabolism in men: current concepts and controversies. *J Endocrinol*. 2014;220(3):R37-R55.

p. 53 *Studies show us that men* ... Pinkhasov RM, Wong J, Kashanian J, et al. Are men shortchanged on health? Perspective on health care utilization and health risk behavior in men and women in the United States. *Int J Clin Pract*. 2010;64(4):475– 487. doi: 10.1111/j.1742–1241.2009.02290.x. Review.

p. 55 *Peer support can help* ... Mathew R, Gucciardi E, De Melo M, Barata P. Self-management experiences among men and women with type 2 diabetes mellitus: a qualitative analysis. *BMC Fam Pract*. 2012;13:122.

p. 57 *Diabetes doubles the risk of depression* ... Anderson RJ, Freedland KE, Clouse RE, Lustman PJ: the prevalence of comorbid depression in adults with diabetes: a meta-analysis. *Diabetes Care*. 2001;24:1069–1078.

p. 57 *Men are less likely to express* … National Alliance on Mental Illness. Depression and men. http://www.nami.org/Template. cfm?Section=Depression&Template=/ContentManagement/ ContentDisplay.cfm&ContentID=88881. Accessed February 8, 2015.

p. 57 *Try drizzling vinegar* … Petsiou EI, Mitrou PI, Raptis SA, Dimitriadis GD. Effect and mechanisms of action of vinegar on glucose metabolism, lipid profile, and body weight. *Nutr Rev*. 2014;72(10):651–661.

p. 57 *You may need to discontinue* … Thomsen HS, Morcos SK, Almén T, et al. Metformin and contrast media. *Radiology*. 2010;256(2):672–673.

p. 58 *Try to avoid these drinks* … Olateju T, Begley J, Green DJ, Kerr D. Physiological and glycemic responses following acute ingestion of a popular functional drink in patients with type 1 diabetes. *Can J Diabetes*. 2015;39(1):78–82.

p. 59 *There have been recent studies* … Siri-Tarino PW, Sun Q, Hu FB, Krauss RM. Meta-analysis of prospective cohort studies evaluating the association of saturated fat with cardiovascular disease. *Am J Clin Nutr*. 2010;91(3):535–546.

p. 59 *It raises LDL* … Lichtenstein AH. Dietary trans fatty acids and cardiovascular disease risk: past and present. *Curr Atheroscler Rep*. 2014;16(8):433.

Chapter 7

p. 66 *Recent studies link diet soda* … Nettleton JA, Lutsey PL, Wang Y, Lima JA, Michos ED, Jacobs DR Jr. Diet soda intake and risk of incident metabolic syndrome and type 2 diabetes in the Multi-Ethnic Study of Atherosclerosis (MESA). *Diabetes Care*. 2009;32(4):688–694.

p. 66 *Recent studies link diet soda* … Gardener H, Rundek T, Markert M, Wright CB, Elkind MS, Sacco RL. Diet soft drink consumption is associated with an increased risk of vascular events in the Northern Manhattan Study. *J Gen Intern Med*. 2012;27(9):1120–1126.

p. 66 *More research is needed, but scientists believe* … Green E, Murphy C. Altered processing of sweet taste in the brain of diet soda drinkers. *Physiol Behav*. 2012;107(4):560–567.

p. 70 *Some research indicates that the anti-inflammatory agents* … Seymour EM, Lewis SK, Urcuyo-Llanes DE, et al. Regular tart cherry intake alters abdominal adiposity, adipose gene transcription, and inflammation in obesity-prone rats fed a high fat diet. *J Med Food*. 2009;12(5):935–942.

p. 70 *Some research indicates that the anti-inflammatory agents* ... Traustadóttir T, Davies SS, Stock AA, et al. Tart cherry juice decreases oxidative stress in healthy older men and women. *J Nutr*. 2009;139(10):1896–1900.

Chapter 8

p. 74 *Recent studies suggest probiotics* ... Gomes AC, Bueno AA, de Souza RG, Mota JF. Gut microbiota, probiotics and diabetes. *Nutr J*. 2014;13:60.

p. 74 *You may need additional immunizations* ... Centers for Disease Control and Prevention. http://www.cdc.gov/vaccines/adults/rec-vac/health-conditions/diabetes.html Accessed February 4, 2015.

p. 75 *Not only does it give you the opportunity* ... Berge JM, Wall M, Larson N, Forsyth A, Bauer KW, Neumark-Sztainer D. Youth dietary intake and weight status: healthful neighborhood food environments enhance the protective role of supportive family home environments. *Health Place*. 2014;26:69–77.

p. 75 *Not only does it give you the opportunity* ... Berge JM, MacLehose RF, Loth KA, Eisenberg ME, Fulkerson JA, Neumark-Sztainer D. Family meals. Associations with weight and eating behaviors among mothers and fathers. *Appetite*. 2012;58(3):1128–1135.

p. 77 *Blueberry consumption* ... Wedick NM, Pan A, Cassidy A, et al. Dietary flavonoid intakes and risk of type 2 diabetes in US men and women. *Am J Clin Nutr*. 2012;95(4):925–933.

p. 77 *Blueberries have also lowered* ... Takikawa M, Inoue S, Horio F, Tsuda T. Dietary anthocyanin-rich bilberry extract ameliorates hyperglycemia and insulin sensitivity via activation of AMP-activated protein kinase in diabetic mice. *J Nutr*. 2010;140(3):527–533.

p 78 *As consumers, we tend to underestimate* ... Wansink B. Environmental factors that increase the food intake and consumption volume of unknowing consumers. *Annu Rev Nutr*. 2004;24:455–479.

p. 78 *In addition, the larger the portions get* ... Wansink, B, Chandon P. Meal size, not body size, explains errors in estimating the calorie content of meals. *Ann Intern Med*. 2006;145(5):326–332.

p. 79 *If you are taking insulin at night* ... Süsstrunk H, Morell B, Ziegler WH, Froesch ER. Insulin absorption from the abdomen and the thigh in healthy subjects during rest and exercise: blood glucose, plasma insulin, growth hormone, adrenaline and noradrenaline levels. *Diabetologia.* 1982;22(3):171–174.

p. 80 *In addition to feeling great* ... Supa'at I, Zakaria Z, Maskon O, Aminuddin A, Nordin NA. Effects of Swedish massage therapy on blood pressure, heart rate, and inflammatory markers in hypertensive women. *Evid Based Complement Alternat Med.* 2013;2013:171852. doi: 10.1155/2013/171852. Epub 2013 Aug 18.

p. 80 *And studies show that it can improve* ... Castro-Sánchez AM, Moreno-Lorenzo C, Matarán-Peñarrocha GA, Feriche-Fernández-Castanys B, Granados-Gámez G, Quesada-Rubio JM. Connective tissue reflex massage for type 2 diabetic patients with peripheral arterial disease: randomized controlled trial. *Evid Based Complement Alternat Med.* 2011;2011:804321. doi: 10.1093/ecam/nep171. Epub 2011 Mar 13.

Chapter 9

p. 84 *Sourdough bread* ... Mofidi A, Ferraro ZM, Stewart KA, et al. The acute impact of ingestion of sourdough and whole-grain breads on blood glucose, insulin, and incretins in overweight and obese men. *J Nutr Metab.* 2012;2012:184710. doi: 10.1155/2012/184710.

p. 85 *Did you know that studies* ... Jyotsna VP. Prediabetes and type 2 diabetes mellitus: evidence for effect of yoga. *Indian J Endocrinol Metab.* 2014;18(6):745–749.

p. 86 *A Duke University study* ... Surwit RS, van Tilburg MA, Zucker N, et al. Stress management improves long-term glycemic control in type 2 diabetes. *Diabetes Care.* 2002;25(1):30–34.

p. 87 *If you are experiencing* ... Feinkohl I, Aung PP, Keller M, et al. Severe hypoglycemia and cognitive decline in older people with type 2 diabetes: the Edinburgh type 2 diabetes study. *Diabetes Care.* 2014;37(2):507–515.

p. 87 *Brain-stretching word games* ... Ferreira N, Owen A, Mohan A, Corbett A, Ballard C. Associations between cognitively stimulating leisure activities, cognitive function and age-related cognitive decline. *Int J Geriatr Psychiatry.* 2014.

p. 88 *The American Diabetes Association recommends ...* American Diabetes Association. 4. Foundations of care: education, nutrition, physical activity, smoking cessation, psychosocial care, and immunization. *Diabetes Care.* 2015;38(suppl. 1):S20-S30. Review.

p. 89 *Studies show coffee ...* O'Keefe JH, Bhatti SK, Patil HR, DiNicolantonio JJ, Lucan SC, Lavie CJ. Effects of habitual coffee consumption on cardiometabolic disease, cardiovascular health, and all-cause mortality. *J Am Coll Cardiol.* 2013;62(12):1043–1051. doi: 10.1016/j.jacc.2013.06.035. Epub 2013 Jul 17. Review.

Chapter 10

p. 93 *It also promotes satiety ...* Flood JE, Rolls BJ. Soup preloads in a variety of forms reduce meal energy intake. *Appetite.* 2007;49(3):626–634. Epub 2007 Apr 14.

p. 94 *A half cup of cabbage ...* Ware M. What are the health benefits of cabbage? *Med News Today.* 2014. Retrieved from http://www.medicalnewstoday.com/articles/284823.php. Accessed January 2, 2015.

p. 95 *In addition, the acetic acid ...* Ostman E, Granfeldt Y, Persson L, Björck I. Vinegar supplementation lowers glucose and insulin responses and increases satiety after a bread meal in healthy subjects. *Eur J Clin Nutr.* 2005;59(9):983–988.

p. 95 *In addition, the acetic acid ...* Johnston CS, Kim CM, Buller AJ. Vinegar improves insulin sensitivity to a high-carbohydrate meal in subjects with insulin resistance or type 2 diabetes. *Diabetes Care.* 2004;27(1):281–282.

p. 97 *And make sure you get ...* Revell VL, Eastman CI. How to trick mother nature into letting you fly around or stay up all night. *J Biol Rhythms.* 2005;20(4):353–365.

p. 98 *Remember, al dente pasta ...* Kirpitch AR, Melinda DM. The 3 R's of glycemic index: recommendations, research, and the real world. *Clin Diabetes.* 2011;29(4):155–159.

p. 99 *There is also some animal research ...* Yoshinari O, Sato H, Igarashi K. Anti-diabetic effects of pumpkin and its components, trigonelline and nicotinic acid, on Goto-Kakizaki rats. *Biosci Biotechnol Biochem.* 2009;73(5):1033–1041. Epub 2009 May 7.

Chapter 11

p. 108 *Studies have shown that if planned correctly* ... Yokoyama Y, Barnard ND, Levin SM, Watanabe M. Vegetarian diets and glycemic control in diabetes: a systematic review and meta-analysis. *Cardiovasc Diagn Ther.* 2014;4(5):373–382.

p. 109 *When reheating* ... United States Department of Agriculture. *Food Safety Fact Sheets: Leftovers and Food Safety.* Available at: http://www.fsis.usda.gov/wps/portal/fsis/topics/food-safety-education/get-answers/food-safety-fact-sheets/safe-food-handling/leftovers-and-food-safety/ct_index. Accessed February 12, 2015.

p. 109 *Did you know that chronic stress* ... Sominsky L, Spencer SJ. Eating behavior and stress: a pathway to obesity. *Front Psychol.* 2014;5:434.

Chapter 12

p. 115 *Some research shows that green tea* ... Liu CY, Huang CJ, Huang LH, Chen IJ, Chiu JP, Hsu CH. Effects of green tea extract on insulin resistance and glucagon-like peptide 1 in patients with type 2 diabetes and lipid abnormalities: a randomized, double-blinded, and placebo-controlled trial. *PLoS ONE.* 2014;9(3):e91163.

p. 115 *Some research shows that green tea* ... Liu K, Zhou R, Wang B, et al. Effect of green tea on glucose control and insulin sensitivity: a meta-analysis of 17 randomized controlled trials. *Am J Clin Nutr.* 2013;98(2):340–348.

p. 116 *Behavioral research has shown* ... Wansink, B, Chandon P. Can "low fat" nutrition labels lead to obesity? *J Mark Res.* 2006;43(4):605–617.

p. 116 *Substances such as ascorbic acid* ... Ginsberg BH. Factors affecting blood glucose monitoring: sources of errors in measurement. *J Diabet Sci Technol (Online).* 2009;3(4):903–913.

p. 117 *One study found that cranberries* ... Lee IT, Chan YC, Lin CW, Lee WJ, Sheu WH. Effect of cranberry extracts on lipid profiles in subjects with type 2 diabetes. *Diabet Med.* 2008;25(12):1473–1477.

p. 118 *Some research indicates that chia ...* Mohd Ali N, Yeap SK, Ho WY, Beh BK, Tan SW, Tan SG. The promising future of chia, *Salvia hispanica* L. *J Biomed Biotechnol*. 2012;2012:171956. doi: 10.1155/2012/171956. Epub 2012 Nov 21. Review.

p. 119 *If you are having unpleasant side effects ...* McCulloch DK. Metformin in the treatment of adults with type 2 diabetes mellitus. In: UpToDate, Nathan DM (Ed), UpToDate, Waltham, MA. Accessed February 3, 2015.

Index

adhesive capsulitis, 117
aerobic exercise, 19, 36, 39. *See also* exercise
air travel, 118. *See also* travel tips
alcohol consumption, 13, 26, 33, 69–70, 117, 120
allergies, 47, 88
almond flour, 98, 107
almond milk, 118
American Diabetes Association (ADA), 18, 106
American Heart Month, 11
anxiety, 5, 15, 44, 46
arterial disease, 80
athletic footwear, 27, 33, 35. *See also* shoes
autonomic neuropathy, 28. *See also* neuropathy

bacterial growth, 7–8, 96
baking tips, 107, 113–115
barbecue grilling, 75
basal insulin, 66
beef, 87
beer, 69–70
bento boxes, 85
blood, donating, 67
blood pressure, 3, 24
blood samples, 16
blood sugar
    chronic infections and, 96
    cold medicines and, 23
    controlling, 3–5, 13, 19, 95
    exercise for, 19
    "15–15 rule," 59
    heat and, 63
    illnesses and, 23, 29, 53, 88

injuries and, 6, 23, 29, 53, 55, 73–77, 80
ketones and, 23
logging, 36
menopause and, 45–46
spike in, 6–7, 57, 79, 95, 117
testing, 3, 6–8, 56, 59, 96, 107, 116
tracking apps for, 96
blood sugar meters, 13, 28, 43–44, 58, 66–69, 89
blood thinners, 94
bloodstains, 97
bolus insulin, 66
bone health, 56, 84–85
bovine insulin, 67
breads, 9, 34, 83–84, 99
breakfasts, 20, 44, 85, 88, 89, 96
buffets, 104
bug bites, 65

calories, burning, 38, 93–94
calories, cutting, 5
cancer risks, 30
candy, 95, 96, 100
carbohydrates. *See also* 15–15 rule
    in casseroles, 35
    counting, 10, 14
    impact of, 7
    lowering, 13
    "net," 67
    "total," 7
cardiovascular disease, 7–8, 11, 14–15, 59
cauliflower comfort foods, 13, 38
celiac disease, 48
certified diabetes educator (CDE), 10, 27, 58, 83

About the Authors

Susan Weiner

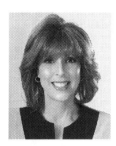

Susan Weiner is owner of Susan Weiner Nutrition, PLLC, in New York. She is an award-winning author, registered dietitian-nutritionist, and certified diabetes educator. Susan is the 2015 AADE Diabetes Educator of the Year and the 2014 Alumna of the Year for SUNY Oneonta. She is also the 2015–2016 editor for *On the Cutting Edge,* a peer-reviewed journal for the Diabetes Care and Education practice group of the Academy of Nutrition and Dietetics. Susan advises several nonprofit groups devoted to diabetes advocacy; she is on the advisory board of Diabetes Sisters, and is an educational advisor for Marjorie's Fund. She is also the diabetes medical advisor for Healthline.com and is on the medical advisory board for dLife. Susan has a master's degree in applied physiology and nutrition from Columbia University in New York and holds a certificate of training in adult weight management through the Academy of Nutrition and Dietetics. You can learn more about Susan and her work at www.susanweinernutrition.com.

Paula Ford-Martin

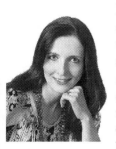

Paula Ford-Martin is an award-winning health writer, editor, and content producer. She is the author of more than a dozen consumer health and parenting books, and currently works as a freelance content strategist and consultant. Paula was part of the core team that created and launched dLife, a groundbreaking multimedia diabetes consumer resource. She served as the Chief Content Officer of dLife for eight years, and her work on CNBC's *dLifeTV*—the first and longest running primetime diabetes television show—garnered her 26 Telly Awards. Paula has a BA in broadcast communications from Marquette University and an MA in writing from DePaul University. She lives in Old Saybrook, Connecticut, with her husband and four children. You can learn more about Paula and her work at www.wordcrafts.com.